"Few medical writers can take complicated scientific material and transform it into a refreshing, stimulating, and easily-read book. Kudos for Dr. Sahelian. He has done a great service to the public hungry for accurate information about this natural supplement. I recommend *Melatonin: Nature's Sleeping Pill* to everyone. Give a copy to your doctor."
Lou Mancano, M.D., Associate Director, Montgomery Hospital Family Practice Residency Program, Norristown, PA

"Anybody middle-aged or older would be well advised to consider melatonin not only for a good night's sleep, but enhanced alertness the next day, better health over the long run, and possibly increased longevity in the bargain. Congratulations to Dr. Sahelian for competently covering such an important topic."
Steven Wm. Fowkes, Executive Director, Cognitive Enhancement Research Institute, Menlo Park, CA; co-author, Smart Drugs II; *Editor,* Smart Drug News

"You have beautifully combined style and substance. *Melatonin: Nature's Sleeping Pill* is a pleasant union of science, clinical experience, and personal stories. You offer excellent information not only to the public, but to physicians, nutritionists, and anyone interested in life extension."
Arnold Fox, M.D., bestselling author of The Beverly Hills Medical Diet *and* The Healthy Prostate Program

"I learned a lot! *Melatonin* is a 'must-read' for anyone who plans to take this natural supplement, or any physician who treats patients suffering from insomnia."
David Schechter, M.D., Clinical Assistant Professor, Department of Family Medicine, University of Southern California School of Medicine, Los Angeles, CA

i

"This book is a masterful blend of raw science, medical journalism, and personal anecdotes. Dr. Sahelian has made an illuminating contribution to mind-body and natural medicine. *Melatonin: Nature's Sleeping Pill* is not only a pleasure to read, but inspiring."
Allen Green, M.D., Medical Director, Institute for Holistic Treatment and Research, Newport Beach, CA

"What a compact mine of fascinating information! *Melatonin* presents the reader with the results of Dr. Sahelian's intensive research into this intriguing substance. Well-balanced, comprehensive, yet fast-reading, *Melatonin* belongs on the shelf of anyone interested in optimum health."
Max More, Ph.D., President, Extropy Institute

"The possibility that melatonin could increase lifespan is fascinating. This book cites legitimate research to support this view. Melatonin is destined to become a household word. As this natural supplement's interesting nature continues to be revealed, we can expect Dr. Sahelian to serve as a reliable interpreter of the ongoing studies."
D. S. Weinstein, M.D., private practitioner, Torrance, CA

"Are you interested in the possibility of a significantly longer, healthier life? Or just in sleeping more easily and soundly at night? In *Melatonin: Nature's Sleeping Pill*, Dr. Ray Sahelian shows us that both may very well be possible, now. The evidence is presented in a clear way for the general reader, and includes extensive references to the scientific literature for the technically inclined. Dr. Sahelian takes care to discuss all known dangers and precautions along with the advantages of supplemental use of this 'wonder' hormone. *Melatonin: Nature's Sleeping Pill* is 'must' reading for all of us interested in better health and greater longevity."

Jonathan V. Wright, M.D., Kent, Washington
Best-selling author of Healing With Nutrition

"A most useful handbook for those needing to improve sleep. *Melatonin: Nature's Sleeping Pill* provides a concise summary of the latest studies with suggestions of possible health benefits through supplementation. A must for melatonin users, prescribers and the sleep deprived."

Priscilla Slagle, M.D., Encino, CA, author of The Way Up From Down

"I read it cover to cover on the plane from LA to Chicago. I found your writing to be focused – not bogged down by irrelevant minutiae. What really made *Melatonin: Nature's Sleeping Pill* enjoyable was the brilliant merging of interesting case histories along with the rigorous scientific data. What otherwise could have been complicated reading turned into a lively and delightful experience."

Christopher B. Heward, Ph.D., endocrinologist; Research Director, Emerald Laboratories, Inc., Carlsbad, CA

"The beneficial potential of melatonin is becoming quickly apparent. There is bound to be a rising flood of controversy between those who would tend to gain or lose from melatonin's growing popularity.

"How timely and fortunate that Ray Sahelian, M.D., has evaluated the pros and cons of this fascinating substance and presented the information in a reader-friendly book. I, for one, fully appreciate Dr. Sahelian's integrity, objectivity, and scientific methodology."

G. Hopkins Schell, M.D., Los Angeles, CA

MELATONIN

NATURE'S SLEEPING PILL

Ray Sahelian, M.D.

Melatonin
Nature's Sleeping Pill

Published by   Be Happier Press
PO Box 12619
Marina Del Rey, CA 90295

Printed in the United States of America
Desktop Publishing by TMS/Russell Kurtz, Ph.D., RussTMS@lamg.com
Illustrations of pineal and prostate by Elise Graham, medical artist.

Sahelian, Ray
    Melatonin: nature's sleeping pill / Ray Sahelian.
    p. cm.
    Includes bibliographical references and index.
    ISBN 0-9639755-7-9
    LCCN 95-094058

    1. Melatonin. 2. Insomnia. I. Title.

    QP572.M44S34 1995   574.1'924
                            QBI95-20018

    ©1995 Be Happier Press

First printing   April 1995   3,000 copies
Second printing   June 1995   20,000 copies   revised and updated

Warning— Disclaimer
    The author, publisher, endorsers, distributors, or anyone else whose name appears in this book shall have neither liability, nor responsibility, to anyone with respect to any loss or damage caused, or alleged to be caused, directly or indirectly by the information contained in this book. Please consult your physician before initiating the use of melatonin or using any sleep-inducing methods mentioned in this book.

Acknowledgments

Thank you for reading the manuscript and offering helpful suggestions.

Cindy Begel, Marina Del Rey, CA

Matthew Brenner, University of California, Santa Cruz

Steve Fechner, Hermosa Beach, CA

Michael Gilbert, President, Albert Hofmann Foundation, who came up with the subtitle

Peter Hauri, *Ph.D.*, director, Mayo Clinic Sleep Disorders Lab, Rochester, Minnesota, for advising on the stages of sleep

Carla Kallan, Culver City, CA

Russell Kurtz, *Ph.D.*, Culver City, CA

Durk Pearson and *Sandy Shaw*, who emphasized the importance of having a separate and complete section on Cautions

Larry Sharp, Playa Del Rey, CA

Suzanne Taylor, Mighty Companions

I wish to also thank all the survey respondents.

Dedicated

to all the scientists
who have spent sleepless nights
discovering the wonders of melatonin.

About the Author

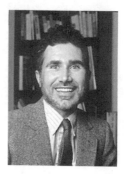

Ray Sahelian, M.D. is a physician certified by the American Board of Family Practice. He obtained a Bachelor of Science degree in nutrition at Drexel University in Philadelphia and completed his doctoral training at Thomas Jefferson Medical School. Following graduation he worked for three years as a resident in family medicine at Montgomery Hospital in Norristown, PA and was involved with all aspects of medical care including pediatrics, cardiology, obstetrics, psychiatry, and surgery.

It was during his residency, with its 36-hour shifts, that he experienced the consequences of sleep deprivation: fatigue, moodiness, and frequent colds. Soon after residency he was employed as a cruise ship doctor for two years in the Caribbean and Hawaii, and caught up on his sleep.

In addition to a medical practice, Dr. Sahelian is a frequent contributor to health magazines; lectures widely on the topics of sleep, health, nutrition, and happiness; and has made numerous appearances on radio and television to discuss his personal experiences with melatonin and the current research now being conducted on this interesting health supplement. He continues to keep a data base of melatonin users from all over the world.

Dr. Ray Sahelian is the author of *Be Happier Starting Now*, a book that has positively influenced many lives.

Author's Note

Melatonin will be big news. It is an effective and inexpensive sleep inducer and word of mouth is rapidly spreading. We have started to understand melatonin's essential role in relation to our immune system, our well-being, and our longevity. We're beginning to understand the full spectrum of melatonin's potential in treating not only sleep disorders, but various other illnesses.

My objective is to introduce the latest research about this extremely intriguing molecule as accurately as possible. Please understand that the clinical use of melatonin is very new.

Medical doctors and scientists have proofread this book, but nothing can be 100% accurate; errors can occur. Please keep this in mind as you are reading the book.

I would like to make it clear that I own no stocks in any company that manufactures, distributes, or retails melatonin. I am a medical doctor and scientist who is objectively presenting the benefits of melatonin, its uncertainties, and its shortcomings.

It is possible to have quality sleep every night. This book will tell you how.

Ray Sahelian, M.D.

Contents

INTRODUCTION

What if there were a safe and natural supplement that in addition to giving you a deep sleep would provide vivid dreams, eliminate jet lag, and also improve your mood? And what if it enhanced your immune system, could treat a variety of diseases, and...even could prolong your life span?

Melatonin, now available without a prescription, may be that very supplement.

A few years ago researchers in Switzerland gave mice melatonin in their drinking water (Maestroni, 1988). Another group of mice received plain water. At the start of the study all the mice were 19 months old (equivalent to about 60 years in humans) and healthy.

The researchers were surprised when the mice on melatonin showed such a striking improvement in their health, and most remarkably, lived so much longer! And after 5 months on melatonin, astonishing differences in the fur quality and vigor of the two groups became evident. The mean survival time of the untreated mice was 25 months (78 years in humans) versus 31 months (98 years) in the melatonin-treated group!

I came across this astounding journal article while doing research at the UCLA biomedical library for my first book, *Be Happier Starting Now*. Since then I have been fascinated by melatonin. My interest peaked even more in 1993, when I learned that it was available to the public over-the-counter, easily purchased off the shelves of the local health food or drug store.

I have researched hundreds of journal articles from all over the world to bring to you the very latest information on this intriguing substance. I personally have taken melatonin supplements in varying doses for one year. I have recommended it to my patients who suffer from insomnia. I have conducted several surveys to collect information from users of melatonin. This book will tell you what I have discovered.

Ray Sahelian, M.D.

ONE

MELATONIN
A SUPPLEMENT FOR THE FUTURE?
OR TONIGHT?

Sleep like a baby.
Improve your mood.
Have more energy.
See vivid dreams.
Prevent jet lag.
And possibly live longer.

What on earth can do all this?

"I've heard of it," said a friend of mine when I told her that I was writing a book on melatonin. "That's skin pigment, isn't it?"

She was thinking of *melanin*, the dark color in skin and hair. Since that conversation I've encountered many people who confuse the two words. Melatonin is a natural hormone made by the *pineal gland*, which is located in the brain (see figure). All words in italics are defined in the glossary.

Melatonin helps to set and control the internal clock that governs the natural rhythms of the body. Each night the pineal gland produces melatonin which helps us fall asleep. Research about this hormone has been going on since it was discovered in 1958. But it is only in the last few years that much attention has been paid to melatonin. Close to a thousand articles a year about melatonin are now published worldwide. One reason for this growing interest is

I

that we are realizing that deep sleep is not the only byproduct of melatonin. We are learning that it has a significant influence on our hormonal, immune, and nervous systems. Research is showing melatonin's role as a powerful *antioxidant*, its anti-aging benefits, and its immune-enhancing properties. It is an effective tool to prevent or cure jet lag, an ideal supplement to reset the biological clock in shift workers, and a great medicine for those who have insomnia. Melatonin also may have a role to play in the treatment of *prostate* enlargement, as an addition to cancer treatment, in lowering cholesterol levels, in influencing reproduction, and more. A delightful bonus is that melatonin can promote vivid dreams.

With all these potential influences on our hormonal and immune systems, no wonder melatonin has been clouded by controversy.

A Controversy That's Bound to Grow

Melatonin supplements became available in health food stores in 1993. Heavy media attention, including CBS, CNN, and major newspaper coverage, was focused on melatonin when a study by MIT researchers, published in March of 1994, showed that it was an effective sleep inducer. Melatonin sales skyrocketed. However, the chief researcher who had directed the study, Dr. Wurtman, sent a letter to the press and appeared on CNN to caution consumers, "I hope that melatonin will become an approved drug quickly. Meanwhile no one should buy it and self-medicate." He argued that there are no agreed-upon dosages, no controls over its purity, and no formal data demonstrating that melatonin is safe. Melatonin sales slumped. The media coverage slowed.

Shortly after this warning, the National Nutritional Foods Association (NNFA), on April 11, 1994, issued an Action Alert to its members: "The leading suppliers and distributors of melatonin products in our industry will be discontinuing distribution of melatonin to health food stores. NNFA agrees with them that mela-

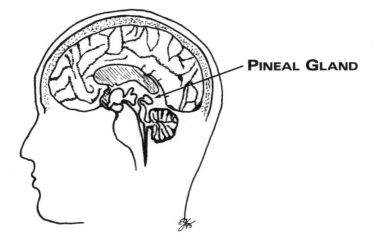

PINEAL GLAND

tonin may be inappropriate as a product to be sold in health food stores and urges retailers to seriously consider the propriety of its continued sale." Nervous health food store managers took melatonin off the shelves (*Whole Foods*, June 1994). It became more difficult for consumers to purchase melatonin. Many relied on mail order distributors for their supply.

The *Wall Street Journal*, in an article published in August 31, 1994, and titled *Drug Companies and Health Food Stores Fight to Peddle Melatonin to Insomniacs*, pointed out, "Dr. Wurtman's letter didn't mention his financial interest in melatonin. Last year he applied for a patent with MIT on the use of melatonin to treat sleep disorders. In March a small Lexington, Mass., company called Interneuron Pharmaceuticals Inc., obtained rights to the patent application. Dr. Wurtman co-founded Interneuron in 1988 and owns nearly one million shares, currently worth about six million dollars. Today, Interneuron is aggressively pursuing a plan to market melatonin as a prescription sleeping pill. The company still faces four or five years of clinical trials, but it thinks it has a long shot at a blockbuster drug." Health food stores would be Interneuron's major competition.

Over the past year, melatonin has started, gradually and quietly, to make a comeback on the shelves of health food and drug stores. Countless individuals have been using melatonin. Word of mouth is rapidly spreading. The controversy is bound to resurface. The news media is starting to pay attention to melatonin again. *Vogue* magazine published an article on melatonin for the use of jet lag in its February, 1995, issue. *Muscle and Fitness* discussed melatonin in its March, 1995, issue.

Major health newsletters have started to voice their opinions about melatonin. The *Johns Hopkins Health After 50* newsletter had an article in its February, 1995, issue, titled *Melatonin: Sleep Aid of the Future?* Their conclusion was, "The research to date on melatonin is encouraging, but it is still too early to consider taking the hormone for sleep disturbances...However, there is no doubt that melatonin plays a role in controlling the sleep/wake cycle, and it is even possible that melatonin will become a useful agent for sleep therapy in the future."

The *University of California at Berkeley Wellness Letter*, in its April, 1995, issue, informed, "So far, at least, there have been no reports of melatonin causing any serious side effects." But the article continued in a tone surprisingly biased. The authors mentioned their concern that supplements sold in health food stores are unregulated and potential contamination can occur. This is true, yet even medicines approved by the FDA have in some cases been found to be contaminated, or have serious health risks. The food we eat can be contaminated. The Agriculture Department estimates 5 million cases of illness and more than 4,000 deaths may be associated with meat and poultry products each year (*Los Angeles Times*, February 1, 1995). As far as I know, neither of the above two medical establishments has discouraged the public from buying vitamins and minerals over-the-counter for fear of contamination. In fact, the *Berkeley Wellness Letter* encourages the public to take vitamins C and E, and calcium supplements. Nor have these institutions discouraged the public from eating chicken. Why raise the contamination issue expressly with melatonin and unnecessarily alarm the public? Having advanced this concern, the authors try to further scare the reader, "Human hormones are powerful substances and can produce unexpected results in long-term use, or even in single large doses." This statement is also true of aspirin, estrogen, prescription sleeping pills, and practically every medicine. Having raised these panic-provoking objections, and with no solid clinical or scientific reasoning to back up their position, the authors conclude, "Don't be a guinea pig. At present we do not recommend that you take it."

I was unsettled after reading this article. I subscribe to this newsletter and have generally found the articles to not only be of high quality, but to present a moderate and objective viewpoint when dealing with complex nutritional issues. If I hadn't researched the scientific studies and done clinical surveys on melatonin myself, I would not have challenged their conclusion.

You will be exposed to various opinions from researchers, medical institutions, physicians, companies, and organizations regarding melatonin's effectiveness and safety. As you formulate your decision on whose opinion to follow, please consider the following factors:

- Is their opinion backed up by solid research? Do they list references?

- Have they done any clinical surveys before formulating their conclusions?

- Will they tend to financially gain or lose from melatonin becoming more popular?

- Does the institution or organization providing an opinion have any financial connections, or friendly relations, with big drug companies that sell prescription sleeping pills?

Hundreds of millions of dollars are spent each year on prescription and over-the-counter sleeping pills. Melatonin could potentially divert a great sum of money from the coffers of pharmaceutical companies who sell sleeping pills to the bank accounts of melatonin manufacturers, distributors, and retailers. It is possible that some claims about melatonin's health benefits are exaggerated. Also possible is that misinformation about its safety is rumored in order to alarm the consumer.

Do not assume that an opinion from a major medical center—or me, or any other physician, researcher, or organization—is gospel. For instance, the *Johns Hopkins* and *Berkeley Wellness Newsletter* articles didn't mention a word about the effect of melatonin on dreams, nor of the studies that found life span extension in rodents when given melatonin. This makes me wonder how much clinical experience the authors really had with melatonin and how much time they spent reviewing research articles. Having worked and studied in renowned hospitals, I know from first-hand experience that some of the physicians who write opinions on particular issues don't necessarily have the needed time to fully read hundreds of articles before formulating their conclusions. They have hospital rounds to perform, lectures to present, meetings to preside over, other types of research to conduct, and recommendations to make on various other medicines and medical illnesses. Furthermore, academics are often insulated from the practical side of day-to-day office medicine. Large institutions are also very cautious and conservative about making new recommendations. Being overcautious by not recommending the use of a safe sleep supplement can be a disservice to the public when the alternative sleep medicines themselves are known to have serious, and potentially fatal, side effects. Patients taking pharmaceutical sleep aids have been known to experience loss of memory and psychosis. Seizures have occurred upon withdrawal.

Throughout this book I will present the benefits of melatonin, its uncertainties, and its shortcomings. As I mentioned in the Author's Note, I do not own stocks in any company. I will not be mentioning or recommending any specific product names or company names. My opinion is based solely on the scientific research, my clinical experience, and the results of my surveys.

I have treated a number of my patients who have insomnia with melatonin. I have conducted various surveys on the internet of melatonin users from all over the country. I have asked everyone I know to notify anyone they know who has used melatonin to call or write to me about their experience. At the time I wrote this book, I had collected information from over 200 users. This number continues to grow daily. If you have used melatonin, please write to me about your experience at the publisher's address listed in the back of the book.

Is Melatonin Effective?

Based on the information I have gathered thus far in my surveys, I have found that about 80% of all survey respondents like the sleep-promoting effects of melatonin and would use it again if needed. About 15% of takers did not feel a significant effect or felt it was too weak for them as a sleep aid, and about 5% have not had a good experience with melatonin and do not wish to try it again.

Is Melatonin Safe?

Whenever researchers want to test the dangers of a substance they give it to laboratory animals such as mice. They give progressively higher and higher doses of the substance until a lethal dose (LD) is reached where 50% of the test animals die. This level is called the LD 50. Back in 1967, at the National Heart Institute in Bethesda, Maryland, Barchas and his colleagues gave mice 800 milligrams (mg) per kilogram (kg) of body weight of melatonin. The mice exhibited no significant ill effects. The researchers needed to give more to find the LD 50, but they could not concentrate the melatonin any further in the amount of liquid that the mice had to drink. The 800 mg/kg is equivalent to giving an average-sized human over 50,000 mg. No other effective sleep inducer is this safe. As we'll discuss later, most people do well with a nightly dose of 3 mg or less.

When human subjects were given as much as 6000 mg nightly for 1 month, some of them complained of abdominal discomfort (Waldhauser, 1990). These high doses did lead to sleepiness the next day, but only for a few hours. No serious side effects were reported. In a longer-term study using high doses, ovarian function was inhibited (similar to the effect of birth control pills) when women took 300 mg nightly for 4 months (Voordouw, 1992). No other side effects were noted. The researchers speculate that high doses of melatonin could be used as an effective oral contraceptive. In a number of animal studies, long-term supplementation of melatonin at high doses has led to reduction of sex hormones such as testosterone and shrinking of the size of *gonads*.

When 6 healthy males were given 2 mg of melatonin each evening for 2 months, no changes in testosterone or other hormone levels were found (Terzolo, 1990).

Twenty young, healthy volunteers were kept in a sleep laboratory for several consecutive nights and were monitored and subjected to a battery of tests (Waldhauser, 1990). After a few nights of this routine, half of the subjects were given a *placebo* and the other half were given 80 mg of melatonin. Those who received melatonin spent less time in bed falling asleep and had fewer awakenings during the night. There was little or no hangover effect the next morning. In fact, the volunteers seemed to perform better in different mental tests and felt more balanced and active. They had a sensation of well-being and emotional stability. This pleasant feeling lasted several hours.

Unlike the study discussed above that found little hangover effect in patients given 80 mg, I found in my surveys of over 200 melatonin users that grogginess for a few minutes in the morning is common for those who take more than 6 mg. Someone described it as a "fuzzy thinking, lethargic feeling." This can last an hour or so after awakening. Lower doses do not cause this.

The longest user of melatonin that I know is Mark, who is 56 years old. He tells me, "I first started buying melatonin from overseas in 1991 before it became available in the US. I've been using 10 mg every third night or so for 4 years and have not noticed any side effects. If I take melatonin every night it loses some of its effectiveness. I don't notice withdrawal or insomnia on the nights that I don't take it. I used to have chronic insomnia. I think melatonin has allowed me to sleep more, and better. I think that this deeper sleep is strongly anti-aging since inadequate sleep accelerates aging."

Since melatonin is produced naturally, the body has evolved mechanisms to remove excessive amounts. It is *metabolized* by the liver and possibly other organs. No reports of any serious side effects have yet been reported in the medical literature. None of the individuals in my surveys have reported any life-threatening or permanent side effects. All the side effects reported have been minor and have quickly disappeared upon discontinuation. I do want to emphasize that melatonin is a new product on the market. It will take many more years before we fully understand all potential positive and/or negative effects.

No substance on this planet can be guaranteed to be 100% safe. Our drinking water can be contaminated. Pure water can even be fatal if a person consumes enormous amounts at one sitting. No activity we engage in is fully safe either. We take a risk every time we go skiing, get in the car to go to the movie theater, or even walk down a flight of stairs.

My position on the use of melatonin differs from that of Dr. Wurtman, Johns Hopkins, and Berkeley. They feel melatonin should at the present not be used at all. Based on the available clinical and scientific data thus far, I believe there is enough evidence to support the occasional use of melatonin. It is a good alternative to prescription and non-prescription sleeping pills.

Even though melatonin is a very safe supplement for short-term use, and promises to be safe for intermittent, longer-term use in low doses, such as 1 mg or less, it is still important that we follow appropriate cautions until more information is available.

Read this book completely, especially the CAUTION section beginning on page 77, before initiating use.

After reading the following chapters, you, in consultation with your physician, will need to decide whether melatonin is appropriate for your needs and whether both of you feel comfortable with its safety. If your physician is not familiar with melatonin, suggest he or she read this book.

Over the next few years many individuals who have insomnia will be helped by using melatonin. A group most likely to appreciate its effects may be the elderly.

Two

From Cradle to Rocking Chair:
Melatonin Throughout Life

Jack is a 74 year old retired pilot. He is in good health and presently is taking no medicines. He came to my office requesting some sleeping pills.

"It takes me at least twenty minutes, sometimes up to an hour, to fall asleep when I get into bed," he said, looking tired.

"How long has this been going on?" I asked.

"For a few years now. I used to put my head on the pillow and be out like a log. But for the past few years it's been a struggle every night. It's terrible."

I asked him how well he slept when he did sleep. "Do you wake up in the middle of the night?" I inquired.

"At least 5 or 6 times. Two times it's to go to the bathroom to urinate."

I explained to him that at his age waking up twice, or even 3 times or more, to urinate is quite normal. The enlargement of the prostate gland in older men narrows the *urethra* and the bladder can't fully empty. This results in frequent visits to the bathroom. During his annual physical exam 4 months earlier, I'd found Jack's prostate gland to be slightly enlarged. I asked him how he felt during the day.

"When I wake up in the morning, I feel like I haven't rested. I nap during the day and can't seem to stay alert. I have nowhere near the energy I used to."

I suggested he try 3 mg of melatonin an hour before bedtime. He called me 2 days later. I could hear the excitement in his voice.

"I took the melatonin at 10:30 pm. I watched *Cheers*, washed my face, brushed my teeth, and went to bed at 11:30 pm. I don't even remember putting my head on the pillow. I only woke up twice to go to the bathroom. I haven't slept so well in years."

Disturbances in the pattern of sleep are very common in the elderly. Older people usually spend more time in bed but less time asleep (Prinz, 1990). They are more easily disturbed from sleep than the young. They wake up more frequently and have trouble falling back asleep. The consequences of inadequate sleep are easily predictable: daytime fatigue, napping, and low mood. Changes in sleep are often age related, and not due to any medical or psychiatric disorders. Contrary to popular belief, there is no evidence that the need for sleep decreases with age (Czeisler, 1992).

A study was conducted in Israel by Haimov and his associates concerning melatonin levels in the elderly, and was published in the *British Medical Journal* in 1994. The results showed that the quality of sleep in the elderly was proportional to the amount of melatonin secreted by their pineal gland. Elderly patients with insomnia had less melatonin secretion at night, half as much as that of young people. The researchers cautiously concluded, "Melatonin deficiency seems to be a key variable in the incidence of sleep disorders in elderly people, and melatonin replacement therapy may prove beneficial."

As you can see from the following graph, levels of melatonin progressively decrease as we age (adapted from Nair, 1986, Waldhauser, 1988 and 1993, and Kloeden, 1993). Why is this?

Scientists are not sure, but have some hypotheses. Initially it was thought that calcium slowly depositing in the pineal gland was

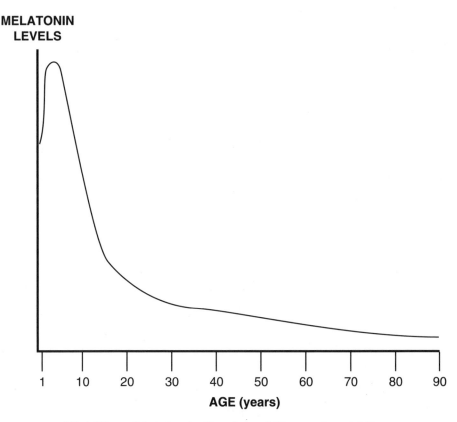

MELATONIN LEVELS

AGE (years)

Nighttime Melatonin Produced Throughout Life.

the culprit. As the gland became calcified, less melatonin was secreted at night. However, a more accepted hypothesis holds that the cells within the pineal gland decrease in number as we age, making it less efficient in producing melatonin (Reuss, 1990).

We sleep roughly 16 hours as infants, 8 hours in adolescence, 7 hours as adults, and less than 6 hours in our geriatric years. Babies up to the age of 3 months don't have well-developed *circadian* rhythms (Jaldo-Alba, 1993). We'll discuss circadian rhythms in detail in Chapter 7. Interestingly, the amount of melatonin in mother's breast milk is dependent upon time of day, with more present at night (Illnerova, 1993). Melatonin, through breast milk, communicates time of day information to babies until they reach 3 months, at which time their circadian rhythm kicks in.

Nighttime melatonin levels peak during early childhood (Waldhauser, 1993). They then drop sharply until early adulthood. This abrupt decrease appears to be due to the continual growth in body size, with the amount of melatonin produced remaining the same. Total melatonin production by the pineal gland then starts decreasing as we age, due to loss of pineal cells. Many people who are past middle age report shallower sleep, since they have less melatonin being produced at night. Interestingly, the release of melatonin in the elderly occurs about an hour earlier at night, which induces older people to go to bed earlier and wake up earlier (Van Coevorden, 1991).

As a tangential note, the sharp decline of melatonin levels in early teen years has been thought to trigger the onset of puberty (Lang, 1984). Administration of melatonin to young experimental animals of both sexes delays puberty (Rivest, 1985).

There are factors besides melatonin depletion that impair the quality of our sleep. These include decreased physical activity, depression, anxiety, illness, medications, menopause, and nocturia (going to the bathroom at night to urinate). Additional causes are listed in Chapter 6.

But remember Jack, the 74 year old retired pilot helped by melatonin? Over the next few months he took melatonin frequently. We found that even 1 mg of melatonin was effective. I encouraged him to take an aerobics class for senior citizens at the local YMCA, and the days he exercised he usually did not need a melatonin supplement at all.

"Doctor, there's something I forgot to mention," added Jack during one of his visits. "I seem to be remembering more dreams than usual. Sometimes they are incredibly vivid."

THREE

DREAMS LIKE YOU'VE NEVER DREAMED

I was holding a bottle of Chianti wine by the neck in my right hand, a walking stick in the other, while hiking through the majestic Dolomite mountains of northern Italy. I slowly meandered up the narrow trail passing granite boulders. Each peek around the bend of a trail opened new vistas of enchanting villages nested in valleys. Soon I reached a narrow, dirt road with low, green hedges on the sides that led to a cobble-stoned plaza of a quaint village. On the left side of the square stood an old gothic church with an arched gate and imposing buttressed walls. Within the square marched a procession of knights. The sun's rays reflected off their silver armor. Behind them followed ladies riding white unicorns. On the right side of the square beckoned a charming outdoor cafe. Each table had a blue and white parasol canopying it. My bottle of wine was empty. I entered the cafe for a refill...and...woke up.

Vivid dreams are common with melatonin use. After experiencing intense dreams myself, and determining through my surveys that many others had experienced the same, I became extremely curious. Throughout the ages humankind has wondered what causes dreams. Many metaphysical explanations have been suggested. Could the answer simply be melatonin? This is what I've learned in my studies and wish to propose as an explanation for the chemicals responsible for dreams.

The chemical name of melatonin is 5-methoxy-N-acetyl-tryptamine (see Appendix). Tryptamines are compounds found abundantly in certain hallucinogenic tropical plants. In South America, Amazonian natives use a form of tryptamine called DMT (N, N-dimethyl-tryptamine), to induce an intense hallucinogenic experience. Some Amazonian shamans use DMT and related hallucinogens for healing purposes and spiritual connections.

When melatonin is metabolized in the pineal gland, it is converted to 5-methoxy-tryptamine (Hardeland, 1993). When rats are given melatonin or 5-methoxy-tryptamine, they spend more time in REM sleep (Mirmiran, 1986), the stage of sleep associated with dreams. It makes sense that melatonin, 5-methoxy-tryptamine, or related tryptamines are involved with dreams. Are there more chemicals involved? We don't know all the answers yet.

We've always thought that hallucinogens were substances foreign to the brain. It is interesting to note that we synthesize natural hallucinogens during sleep; they are a normal part of our brain chemistry. Moreover, our brain does not seem to develop a tolerance to these tryptamine hallucinogens since we dream every night, whether we remember the dreams or not.

In order to find out whether anyone else had come up with the theory that tryptamines were involved with dreams, I placed a question on a few usenet groups on the internet, including sci.life-extension and alt.psychoactives. The post was titled "Melatonin, dreams, and tryptamines." Two days later I got a message from J.C. Callaway, Ph.D., from the University of Kuopio, Finland. He referred me to an article he had published in the journal *Medical Hypotheses* in 1988. Dr. Callaway believes tryptamines and related compounds are the chemicals responsible for dreams.

Throughout my surveys I found that about two out of three respondents had experienced vivid dreams— the higher the melatonin dose, the more likely. David, a 35 year old, says, "I've been taking 3 mg of melatonin for about 5 months— not every night, but perhaps 4 nights a week. I tend not to dream. Recently, I tried 6 mg, and noticed that I do have dreams on this dose."

In my surveys, about 5% of people taking melatonin reported having had bad dreams or nightmares. Melatonin accentuates dreams. If an individual's dreams are usually pleasant, they will continue being so, but more intensely. If dreams are normally unpleasant, then it is possible they will be worse. Pam, a 21 year old student, writes, "I took 3 mg of melatonin. It worked quite fast and I slept fairly soundly except after an awful nightmare. From then on my sleep was restless and I kept waking up. This was the second time I had taken melatonin. The first time I had one particularly vivid dream, and it was okay."

If you recall the diagram in Chapter 2, the highest levels of melatonin are present during early childhood. This is also the time of life when intense pleasant dreams and nightmares occur most frequently. Is this another clue to the puzzle?

In order to reduce the likelihood of unpleasant dreams, develop a positive attitude and good self-esteem. Steer away from negative brain input such as violent TV shows or horror movies. Nurture a loving connection with people, nature, and animals. For a detailed approach to mood improvement and enhancing the quality of life, thus more pleasant dreams, please refer to my book *Be Happier Starting Now.*

If you need to take melatonin for a sleep disorder but do not wish to have vivid dreams or nightmares, take as small a dose as necessary. Low doses, perhaps as little as 0.5 mg, are less likely to intensify dreams.

Whether or not you believe that dreams have meaning (some believe they are simply the random firing of *neurons*), it can be fun to recall these vivid dreams and write them down in a diary soon upon awakening. Even if you can't find meaning in them, they can always make interesting conversation over the breakfast table.

More About Dreams

Over the course of a night adults dream on the average once each 90 minutes (5 to 6 times during the entire night). The duration of these dreams increases over the course of the night, from about 5 to 10 minutes at the end of the first 90 minute sleep cycle, to about 45 minutes at the end of the last. People usually recall their dreams 1 out of every 2 nights. Some users of melatonin find the morning dream lasts extremely long, somewhat like a double feature at the movie theater.

Some psychologists and sleep researchers theorize that dreams reflect our subconscious or conscious hopes, fears, and emotional states. For example: the hope or wish to travel may lead to a dream that involves visiting a foreign country. I have never been to the Dolomite mountains in Italy, but a friend of mine visited there a year ago and raved about them. Perhaps, months later, this influenced my dreams about hiking there. Fear due to an upcoming exam may be expressed in a dream where one finds it impossible to write on the test sheet. There may be no ink in the pen or one's hand may be paralyzed. A person who has been reprimanded for being late at work may have a dream where he is stuck in traffic and all exits are blocked.

Bad dreams are not necessarily bad to have. Some dreams bring up issues we have not adequately addressed during waking hours. Recurrent dreams give us the opportunity to confront and solve problems that we have been avoiding. Dreams also provide us with an opportunity to rehearse solutions to situations that threaten us— an obvious evolutionary advantage. If the intensity of a suppressed emotion is strong enough, the dream may be so intense that it causes us to wake up. This can be a signal by our unconscious mind to focus on this issue and resolve it. Therefore, it is possible that we can learn from bad dreams to see what it is we are repressing. We can then take steps to confront and deal with the issue.

Perhaps psychiatrists who specialize in dream interpretation will take advantage of melatonin's dream-enhancing properties to induce vivid dreams in their patients and thus offer a better opportunity for analysis.

Back to Jack

"There's one more thing I wanted to ask you," said Jack. "I really like the quality of my sleep when I take melatonin. I feel great the next day and notice my mood is better. What would happen if I took melatonin every night?"

I told Jack about some very interesting findings in mice when they were given melatonin for prolonged periods.

FOUR

MELATONIN AND LONGEVITY

Wouldn't it be great if science discovered supplements that could prolong our life span? Perhaps that time is not far away. Perhaps that time is now. Perhaps melatonin is one of these supplements.

Life Span Extension in Animals

In my introduction, I discussed the experiment by Maestroni and colleagues, published in 1988, that found an average 20% increase in longevity in middle-aged, male mice when they were given melatonin in their nightly drinking water. The researchers state, "To our surprise, chronic, nightly administration of melatonin resulted in a progressive, striking improvement of the general state of the mice and, most important, in a remarkable prolongation of their life. In fact, starting at 5 months from the initiation of melatonin administration, the body weight of the untreated mice still surviving started to decrease rapidly, and also astonishing differences in the fur and in the general conditions of the 2 groups (vigor, activity, posture) became increasingly evident. Melatonin treatment preserved completely optimal pelage (fur) conditions."

A similar experiment on middle-aged, male mice, done in 1991 by Pierpaoli and colleagues, also found a 20% increase in life span.

What would melatonin do in the young? To find out, Pierpaoli and colleagues gave melatonin every night to young, female mice (strain C3H/He) starting at age 12 months until death. (There are various strains of laboratory mice and the effect of a particular substance may be different on each strain. That's why it's important to mention which one.) The average life span in this strain of mice is about 24 months. The age of 12 months (pre-menopause) would correspond roughly to age 35 in humans. To the surprise of everyone, melatonin shortened life span by 6%. A high rate of ovarian cancer occurred in these young mice. Apparently there are cells in the ovaries in this strain that overgrow when stimulated by melatonin, causing tumors. Another strain of young, female mice (NZB) was also given melatonin nightly starting at age 12 months, and they lived longer than the untreated group. A third group of NZB strain female mice was given melatonin at 5 months of age (Pierpaoli, 1994). They also lived longer than those not on melatonin. Obviously, different mouse strains respond to melatonin differently.

It is possible that if the mice who developed ovarian cancer had been given a lower dose of melatonin, they may have fared better. Based purely on a weight ratio, the amount of melatonin given the mice was many times the dose a human would normally use at night for sleep.

How did melatonin affect female mice who already had reached menopause? In one study, when 18 month old post-menopausal mice (strain C57BL/6) were given melatonin nightly, ovarian cancer was not detected. They lived 20% longer than those who were not given melatonin.

How can we interpret these animal studies in order to make practical recommendations for us humans? First, we have to realize that rodents and humans may respond differently to the same medicine. We have seen that even different strains of mice respond differently. We know by experience, however, in countless other studies and with various other medicines that there is often a similarity between the effects of a substance on rodents and that on humans. We should also consider the possibility that while one person may benefit from a medicine, another may be harmed. Just as there are differences in response between different strains of mice, there may be differences in response between different human beings.

In order for us to know what melatonin will do in humans when given for a lifetime, we would need to follow hundreds or thousands of people. Multiple groups would be needed to try different dosages. Such a comprehensive study is not under way at this time. Even if it were, the results would not be available until well into the 21st Century. What shall we do in the meantime?

Different scientists familiar with these studies may recommend different courses of action. One scientist may caution, "Let's wait a few more years." Another may advocate, "If we wait, we'll have to wait decades. I'm 65 now and I'm having trouble sleeping at night. Melatonin provides me with great sleep. In addition it could extend my life span." Who will eventually be proved right? No one can be sure at this time.

There are additional studies that support the role of melatonin and the pineal gland in life extension. It has been known for decades that when rodents have their pineal glands removed, they die sooner (Malm, 1959). When the pineal glands of 4 month old mice were transplanted into 18-month-old mice, the older mice lived longer and aging symptoms were postponed (Lesnikov, 1994). When young mice receive the pineal gland from older mice, they die sooner.

The pineal gland releases substances other than just melatonin that play a role in longevity. One such example is epithalamin, which, together with other pineal gland extracts, has produced life extension in mice (Anisimov, 1994).

How Can Melatonin Extend Life Span?

The pineal gland communicates with every cell of the body through its primary hormone, melatonin. Most hormones need a *receptor* on the *cell membrane* before they can enter the cell. Not so for melatonin. As the pineal gland releases melatonin, it quickly goes into the local bloodstream and then into general circulation. From there, melatonin finds its way to every body fluid and tissue. Melatonin has the unusual capacity to easily permeate tissues and enter practically every cell of the body. When melatonin enters the cells, it goes into every compartment, including the nucleus. Researchers speculate that the amount of melatonin reaching the DNA of each cell informs that cell as to which proteins to make. The November 1994 *Journal of Biological Chemistry* reported that researchers Becker-Andre and colleagues found a specific receptor for melatonin right in the nucleus of cells. They conclude, "A nuclear signaling pathway for melatonin may contribute to some of the diverse and profound effects of this hormone."

One theory proposes that during infancy and childhood there is a high level of melatonin reaching every cell. This high level lets the cells know that the organism is young. Proteins necessary for growth and repair are manufactured. The amount of melatonin released each night is lessened in adults and reduced even more in old age. Therefore, as we advance in years, less melatonin reaches the DNA in our cells. Some researchers (Kloeden, 1993) think the pineal gland functions as a centralized clock to coordinate genes switching on and off.

This decline of melatonin levels may inform all cells of the body's age— *i.e.*, it's time to call it quits, call a lawyer, write a living will, and put the first down payment on a cemetery plot (or cryonics arrangements for futurists). Melatonin supplementation could trick the DNA into thinking, "Maybe I miscalculated. I must be younger than I thought."

We should not think of melatonin as the only influence on aging. In a complex organism such as the human body there are countless factors influencing the aging process. The pineal gland is only one of these factors, albeit an important one.

Some of the ways melatonin could prolong life span include its ability to enhance the immune system, regulate hormonal levels, and act as an *antioxidant*. There's also an interesting correlation between diet and melatonin. Food restriction in rodents causes an increase in melatonin production (Stokkan, 1991). Food restriction also leads to their life extension. It is too early to tell whether the increase in melatonin due to food restriction causes this longevity (Huether, 1994).

A Powerful Antioxidant

Many diseases are now believed to be caused or aggravated by free radicals. A free radical is any molecule with an unpaired electron restlessly going around ravaging and harming other molecules—like a hyperactive child swirling around a playpen breaking toys. Free radicals are formed as the end result of burning glucose and other energy molecules within our cells. When we drive a car, we burn gasoline as fuel. The leftovers are spewed out through the tail pipe of the exhaust system. When food is broken down and then metabolized, it similarly creates byproducts. These free radicals are some of the harmful molecules that are left over. They include molecules called hydroxyl ($OH^{\bullet}$), superoxide ($O_2^{\bullet -}$), and hydrogen peroxide (H_2O_2). Hydroxyl radicals are thought to be the most damaging (Reiter, 1994).

In the past few years researchers have found that melatonin possesses unique properties as a free radical neutralizer. Melatonin is not only able to trap free radicals such as superoxide anions, but is also very efficient at preventing damage from hydroxyl radicals. Melatonin has been found to be the most potent neutralizer of hydroxyl radicals ever detected. It stops damage immediately and is more effective as an antioxidant than even vitamins C and E (Hardeland, 1993). It also stimulates the enzyme glutathione peroxidase, which converts destructive hydrogen peroxide, H_2O_2, to safe water, H_2O (Reiter, 1993). Researchers in France have also confirmed melatonin's antioxidant abilities (Pierrefiche, 1993).

Many antioxidant vitamins and nutrients lack the capacity to enter cells and *organelles* as easily as does melatonin. Melatonin has the advantage of being able to freely enter and permeate all parts of a cell. In a study of DNA damage induced by safrole, a cancer promoting agent, melatonin protected the DNA almost entirely from free radical damage (Tan, 1994). This occurred even though melatonin was given at $\frac{1}{1000}$ the dose of the carcinogen. Melatonin also has been found to bind to *chromatin* within the nucleus of a cell, thus indicating that it may have direct on-site protection of DNA. As discussed earlier, melatonin levels decrease as we age. Researchers speculate that lower melatonin levels may not be able to protect brain cells (neurons) from normal wear and tear. Furthermore, the activity of some brain enzymes, such as MAO-B, *monoamine oxidase type B*, can increase with age, leading to more breakdown of neurotransmitters and more free radical production. The failure of neurons and the decline of neurotransmitters may then accelerate, leading to dementia, *Alzheimer's* disease, *Parkinson's* disease, and other degenerative mental illnesses. As Hardeland and associates concluded in their 1993 article, "Melatonin promises to become a powerful pharmacological agent with its unique properties as a nontoxic, highly effective radical scavenger which provides protection eventually from neurodegeneration as well as from the mutagenic and carcinogenic actions of hydroxyl radicals." In other words, melatonin, taken as a supplement, could slow down the aging process and decrease the incidences of brain damage and cancer.

Russell J. Reiter, a highly respected pineal gland researcher at the University of Texas Health Science Center in San Antonio, concluded in a 1994 article published in the *Annals of the New York Academy of Sciences*, "Melatonin may prove to be the most important free radical scavenger discovered to date."

Diseases that may be caused or aggravated by free radical damage include atherosclerosis (blockages in arteries), *emphysema*, cataracts, Parkinson's, *Lou Gehrig's*, other neurological diseases, and some forms of cancer.

Enhancing Immunity

A complicated interaction between our immune system, hormones, and nervous system allows our bodies to adapt to the external world and prevents us from coming down with infections. The pineal gland is intimately involved in regulating these systems. Receptors for melatonin have been found in lymphoid organs such as the thymus and spleen (Poon, 1994) and on white blood cells (Lopez-Gonzalez, 1993).

Melatonin is believed to enhance the immune system. Mice given melatonin had an increased response of *immune globulins* to *antigens* (Maestroni, 1988, Caroleo, 1994). The researchers speculate that vaccines may be more effective when given at the same time as melatonin supplements. Even when mice were given *cortisol*, a substance which depresses the immune system, additional melatonin counteracted the detrimental effects of the cortisol (Maestroni, 1986).

Melatonin counteracts the effects of stress on the immune system. When mice are restrained, their *antibody* production drops, the weight of their *thymus* gland decreases, and their resistance to viruses lessens. Evening administration of melatonin buffered them against the effects of stress (Maestroni, 1988). Many of the harmful effects on the immune system by stress are closely related to signs and symptoms of aging. In the elderly, the thymus gland shrinks and immunity is lowered. Since aging is associated with lower melatonin levels, melatonin replacement may have a role in improving immunity. The elderly are particularly susceptible to pneumonia, flu, and other infections.

Recent studies indicate that melatonin may restore the function of the thymus gland. The thymus gland is involved with the production and maturation of T *lymphocytes*. Melatonin stimulates the production of T lymphocytes in those who have a poorly functioning immune system (Maestroni, 1993). The mineral zinc is also thought to improve the functioning of the thymus gland. Melatonin is believed to facilitate the interaction of zinc with the thymus gland, allowing another pathway of immune enhancement (Mocchegiani, 1994).

Sze and colleagues found that giving mice melatonin for 2 weeks induced production of powerful virus and bacteria fighting substances such as *interferon* and *interleukin-2*.

We all know how great it feels the day after 8 hours of uninterrupted slumber. We feel younger, more energetic, almost forgetting that there is such a thing as "tired." For the elderly who have low melatonin levels, and toss and turn all night, supplementation could provide that refreshing rest so critical to well-being. In an article published in the November/December, 1994, issue of *Psychosomatic Medicine*, Michael Irwin, MD, and colleagues, at the San Diego Veterans Affairs Medical Center, studied 23 healthy men, ages 22 to 61. All spent 4 nights in a sleep laboratory. On the third night, volunteers were denied sleep between the hours of 3 am and 7 am. The majority of the subjects had substantially reduced activity of their white blood cells, specifically *natural killer* (NK) cells. NK cells help protect us from viruses and the abnormal growth of cancer cells.

In brief, melatonin seems to improve the functioning of the immune system by restoring the thymus gland, increasing interferon production, enhancing antibody production, and enhancing anti-tumor factors (Caroleo, 1994).

To Take, or Not to Take: That is the Question

I know a number of individuals who have started taking melatonin nightly at doses ranging from 1 mg to 10 mg. They do not necessarily take melatonin for sleep, but for its potential health and longevity benefits. Four of these individuals have been taking it for over 2 years, with no apparent side effects. Some organizations involved in seeking ways for life extension are recommending that their members use melatonin regularly.

A few pineal gland researchers have started to take melatonin for its potential health benefits. Russel Reiter is quoted in *Vogue*, February, 1995, as saying, "I've been taking it [melatonin] for years for jet lag. When we made the discovery about its antioxidant potential, I started taking it regularly." (He takes about 1 mg nightly.)

As mentioned earlier, we don't know for certain the long-term effects of melatonin use in humans— positive or negative. Then again, we hardly know the long-term effects of many common medicines or supplements, including aspirin and vitamins. However, we do know how melatonin has been used in the short term to help people, as we'll see in Chapter 6. But first, let's look at some practical matters involving dosage and timing.

FIVE

TAKE TWO MELATONINS
AND CALL ME IN THE MORNING

What Dosage is Best?

Melatonin supplements are currently available in 0.2 mg, 0.3 mg, 0.75 mg, 1 mg, 2 mg, 3 mg, 5 mg, and 10 mg pills or capsules. Some bottles list dosages in mcg (micrograms); 1 mg (milligram) equals 1000 mcg. Lozenges, which are dissolved in the mouth, are available in 1 mg, 2 mg, 2.5 mg and 5 mg. Melatonin is not patented, so a number of companies manufacture and distribute it. A wide range of doses works for people. Each person has a unique physiology, hence, no blanket statements about dosages can be made. A person may also require a higher amount during nights when he or she is extremely alert, upset or preoccupied.

Furthermore, the amount of melatonin available in capsules, pills, or lozenges may vary between products and manufacturers. The length of time that a particular bottle is stored may also make a difference. Melatonin is a stable molecule, but its potency could slowly decrease with time. Refrigeration is not necessary, but may help melatonin's potency to last longer.

It may be best to take melatonin on an empty stomach or with a small meal. A melatonin pill taken on a full stomach does not seem to be as consistently effective. This may be because the pill is not fully absorbed, or simply absorbed too slowly. After swallowing a pill, peak levels in the blood are found in about 1 hour. An interesting finding in a previously discussed study referred to in Chapter 1 (Waldhauser, 1984) was that the amount of melatonin absorbed from the digestive system and present in the bloodstream of different volunteers sometimes varied by a factor of 300! This shows the uniqueness of each individual's digestion and absorption.

Melatonin in the range of 0.3 mg to 10 mg is effective in inducing a natural yawn and maintaining a deep sleep in most people. We need to keep in mind that pills or lozenges may not contain exactly the amount specified on the bottle. This is true of any medicine or pill. The production process is not perfect, and not all pills will contain the same exact dose.

If a person fails to respond to a low dose, such as 0.5 mg or 1 mg, a higher dose, such as 2 to 5 mg, may do the trick. If there is no response to pills, lozenges can be tried. Lozenges seem to be more consistently effective than pills since they do not need to be absorbed from the stomach. The melatonin directly enters the bloodstream from absorption through the mouth. Some individuals find that a smaller dose from a lozenge may be as effective as a larger dose from a pill.

There are some people who respond weakly even to high doses. Ted, a 23 year old student, informs me, "I took what I believe was an overdose, two 3 mg pills and two 5 mg lozenges, a total of 16 mg. It did seem to induce in me that sleepy state right before one falls asleep, but the feeling wasn't overwhelming. In fact, I only felt sleepy when I laid on my bed; otherwise I think I could have stayed up longer."

Wayne, a 24 year old computer programmer from Seattle, asserts, "I have severe chronic insomnia and I've used melatonin twice. Neither time did it seem to improve my sleep. (My body is amazingly good at resisting sleep.) Both were 3 mg doses taken just a few minutes before bed."

Keep in mind that melatonin is subtle compared to the effects of prescription sleeping pills. It doesn't have their knockout punch. Matthew, a 25 year old editor, tells me, "I am impressed at the similarity between melatonin and natural sleep. As someone who has suffered periodic bouts of insomnia, melatonin provided natural sleepiness without the drowsiness of some prescription medicines that I've taken in the past." Heather, a 24 year old massage therapist, nods, "Sleep comes on naturally and peacefully."

Some individuals do very well with small doses. A survey respondent wrote, "I'm 57 years old and have been taking melatonin regularly for insomnia for a year. Previously, I would sleep 4 or 5 hours, then wake up and not be able to go back to sleep. With 1.25 mg of melatonin I sleep through the night. If I do happen to wake up, I am able to easily fall back asleep. I've had no side effects at all and wake up refreshed."

For most people melatonin is effective the very first night. However, some may take up to 3 nights before noticing a difference. MacFarlane and colleagues also noted this. "Improved sleep is in evidence from the first treatment night, but an increased efficacy is observed with repeated treatments."

When is the Best Time to Take Melatonin?

People vary widely in their response times. Pills are effective for most people when taken about half an hour to 3 hours before bed. Lozenges dissolved in the mouth seem to work when taken between 20 minutes and 2 hours before going to bed. Most people notice a natural yawn within half an hour of dosing. I, personally, do well with a quarter or even a fifth of a 5 mg lozenge taken 2 hours before bedtime. When I put my head on the pillow, I'm out! I have found that a lower dose is more effective when taken at least 2 hours before bed while a higher dose can be taken closer to bedtime.

One of the most common mistakes people make when dosing with melatonin is taking it too close to bedtime. This is not a prescription sleeping pill and doesn't work as quickly. For the most part, a good 30 minutes to 2 hours is required for best results. And remember: tablets and lozenges from different manufacturers may be absorbed at different rates.

Leona, a 42 year old social worker, told me, "I took a 2.5 mg lozenge right before bed. I didn't feel any effects from it and had trouble falling asleep. I tried it again a few nights later right before bed. Still no effect. I was almost going to give up on melatonin when you suggested I try it at least 1 hour before bed. This seemed to make all the difference; I went to sleep within a couple of minutes of putting my head on the pillow."

One survey respondent wrote that he has chronic insomnia and takes 10 mg of melatonin an hour before bed. He wakes up at 3 or 4 am and takes another 10 mg. This works for him; he feels fine the next day. Another user noted that he once woke up at 3 am and couldn't fall asleep. He hadn't taken any melatonin the night before. After an hour of tossing in bed, he took two 3 mg pills at 4 am and had trouble getting out of bed the next day. He felt groggy most of the morning. The next night he didn't feel sleepy until 3 in the morning. By taking the melatonin in the middle of the night, he had reset his circadian rhythm to a different time. It's best to take melatonin to accentuate the natural sleep rhythm avoiding the use at an odd hour where it could shift the cycle to an undesired time.

One friend has found that breaking a pill in small portions and taking about 0.5 mg 2 hours before bed and taking another 0.5 mg 1 hour before bed gives her a better sleep than taking it all at one time. This is probably a good strategy since melatonin is gradually produced by the pineal gland at night. One could therefore take small doses maybe 3 hours, 2, and 1 hour before bed. I tried this approach recently. I nibbled tiny amounts from a 5 mg lozenge 3 hours before, 2 hours before, and 1 hour before bed. It worked very well. I must have taken a total of less than one fifth of the lozenge.

These anecdotes indicate the importance of trial and error in finding out the best dose and the best time for your unique self.

Is Melatonin Addictive?

Since no studies in humans have yet been published specifically addressing the question of addiction, I can't make a definitive statement about melatonin's addictive potential. I can only state my own experience and the experience of 200 users who feel melatonin not to be physically addictive. Those who take it for its anti-aging effects use it regularly and aren't concerned with addiction. The majority of users who take it for improved sleep only take it when they really need it. A few mentioned that they liked the improved quality of sleep so much that they wanted to use melatonin often— almost like a weak psychological addiction. It is possible that melatonin can be habit forming. Stuart, a regular user for 4 months, is one example: "I don't have a strong urge to take it but I can tell the difference in the quality of my sleep when I do use it. At night, when its getting close to bedtime I sometimes think to myself, you know, I really want to sleep well tonight. So, often I pop a pill."

Dennis, a 52 year old, writes, "I have been a vegetarian and meditator for 20 years. Anything I take routinely I make a practice of not taking for 1 day a week, 1 week per month and 1 month per year. With melatonin I have noticed no withdrawal, no feeling of addiction, and no noticeable effect other than natural restful sleep when I take it. Honestly, it feels like something my body is missing and should have, and welcomes it when I take it. I feel no 'impact' like drugs, pharmaceuticals, or concentrated potions. Great stuff."

For the past year I've taken about 1 mg of melatonin most nights. My sleep has been extremely deep and restful. I recently stopped taking it for a week and have noticed no withdrawal symptoms. My sleep is back to what it was before having started melatonin. When not taking melatonin, I normally sleep 7 hours, waking up once or twice. When I take a melatonin supplement, I sleep about an hour longer, deeper, and rarely wake up. I personally find that there is a slight habit forming tendency, and, as Stuart reported above, it is tempting to use melatonin regularly since the sleep it provides is so soothing.

John, a 44 year old computer technician from San Francisco, does not believe melatonin is addictive. "Not at all. The inverse. Once the body has enough, it seems to be able to use the built up stores. Others at the health food store have commented the same."

Most users find that they sleep half an hour or an hour longer when they take melatonin. A few find they sleep fewer hours, but more efficiently. The majority feel more refreshed and energetic the next day.

What About Tolerance?

No formal studies have been done in humans regarding tolerance to melatonin. The use of most pharmaceutical sleeping medicines is known to lead to tolerance. Higher and higher doses are often needed. Tolerance to melatonin seems to be present, but infrequent. Less than a tenth of my survey respondents felt the need to take higher doses. Jerry, a 67 year old chiropractor from Miami, tells me, "I've been using 1.5 mg of melatonin regularly for 7 months. It seems to be as effective now as the first few nights." Tolerance is even less frequent in those who do not use melatonin every night, but take breaks once in a while.

There are a few people who have noticed that they need a higher dose of melatonin than they used to. Bruce, from San Jose, writes, "I never felt a craving for melatonin, or felt like I couldn't do without it. Three mg worked for me for quite a while, and whether it was a matter of gaining some level of tolerance to it or just the rather substantial (read HUGE) increase in stress in my life, I can't say. I know that 6 mg works now. The tolerance was something that cropped up over a matter of months of casual use."

Personally, I have not noticed any tolerance. One mg is still quite effective to induce and maintain sleep for me, as it was a year ago. I am presently using melatonin 4 or 5 times a week.

Are There Withdrawal Symptoms?

Abruptly stopping prescription sleep medicines after chronic use can often result in sleep disturbances for a week or two. For some it takes longer. Data from my surveys suggest that withdrawal symptoms from the abrupt discontinuation of chronic melatonin use are infrequent, causing only minor and short-lived sleep disturbances. There is little or no insomnia the night following discontinuation, and any disturbances are corrected within a few days.

Steve Dyer, 38, a software engineer from Cambridge, Mass., writes, "I find that melatonin is very effective at helping me get to sleep. Originally, a single lozenge was all that I needed, but I found that 4 lozenges worked better. I go to bed on-time, and wake up on-time, refreshed.

"I used 10 mg of sublingual melatonin, four 2.5 mg lozenges, for several months. Upon stopping it, I had no rebound insomnia at all."

Now that we know some of the practical details of using melatonin, let's see how we can put these to use.

68 - prostate; BPH
70 - osteoporosis, scoliosis
8 - 3 mg or less for sleep

Six

Uses of Melatonin

Evidence continues to accumulate in research journals and case studies about melatonin's effectiveness in treating many conditions. This chapter focuses on those conditions for which the use of melatonin has been well documented. The last chapter of the book will discuss uses of melatonin for which research is in the very early stages.

Insomnia

Up to 40% of adults endure frequent nights of inadequate sleep. As a family physician I often hear from frustrated patients about their difficulties in getting a restful night. When I give lectures or seminars on how to sleep better, countless people describe to me their anguish and despair. One young woman says that even walking past her bedroom gives her a panicky feeling. She fears her bed. She associates her bed with horrible nights of alertness in the dark.

Many insomniacs use over-the-counter medicines like Benadryl, Nyquil, or Sominex. Some try herbal products such as valerian root or sip chamomile tea.

There are many causes for inadequate or disrupted sleep (see the following table). If you suffer from insomnia, consult this list to see if any of the reasons apply to you. Take necessary steps to correct them. Follow the twenty tips to deep sleep as outlined in Chapter 9. If, after following all these steps, you continue with frequent episodes of insomnia, consult a physician to make sure you have no serious medical or psychological causes. If your exam and tests are normal, it may be appropriate to temporarily attempt the help of a sleep medicine. A good choice is melatonin.

MacFarlane, from McMaster University in Toronto, Canada, tested the effect of 75 mg of melatonin administered nightly at 10 pm to 13 insomniacs. A significant improvement in sleep and daytime alertness was observed with melatonin compared to treatment with placebo. Six of the 13 participants also reported improved mood. In some insomniacs the response to melatonin was delayed by several nights.

The dosage used to treat insomnia is quite variable. One option is to start with 1 mg 2 hours before bed. Try this for a few nights. If no improvement is noted, try 2 or 3 mg. Use this higher dosage for a few more nights. Experiment to see what hour before bedtime is right for you to take melatonin. Some people may find taking a pill several hours before bed helps them more than taking it 1 hour before. It may be trial and error until you come up with the best dosage and timing for your unique self.

There is a condition called delayed sleep phase insomnia. People with this condition cannot fall asleep at the same clock time, but have no difficulty sleeping when bedtime is delayed 2-5 hours. If bedtime the first night is 12 midnight, the following night they would sleep normally at 2 am, the night after at 4 am, and so on. Melatonin seems to be very effective for patients who have this syndrome. It resets their clock, by advancing their sleep phase. Dahlitz, from the University of London, successfully treated 8 patients with this syndrome using 5 mg of melatonin at 10 pm.

In cases of severe insomnia where a pharmaceutical pill alone is not effective, combining it and melatonin, both at low doses, may be of great benefit (Ferini-Strambi, 1993). Taking lower doses of pharmaceutical sleeping pills should reduce their side effects.

When deciding to stop the use of melatonin or any sleeping medicine, it is best to taper off over a period of 1 to 2 weeks to avoid any sleep disturbances. Melatonin may in some individuals cause rebound insomnia, as do some other sleeping pills, but to a much lesser degree. Only a small percentage of people feel any withdrawal symptoms. Marilyn, a survey participant, writes, "I stopped taking melatonin last summer after regular use and noticed no withdrawal symptoms at that time. Most recently, I have noticed that if I stop taking it after a few days (usually 3 or 4), I have more trouble falling asleep. I also wake more often during the night."

Jerry, from Denver, notes, "I took 3 mg of melatonin for 2 months because I was going through a rough divorce. I stopped taking it last week and did not notice any withdrawal. My sleep is not as deep, but not any different than what it was before I started taking melatonin."

Even though withdrawal is uncommon, and mild, it is still best to taper off slowly. For example, if you have been using 3 mg of melatonin regularly for a while and you feel you don't need it anymore, lower the dose to 2 mg for a few nights, then 1 mg for another few nights, and stop.

Sleeping problems in children have also been treated successfully with melatonin supplements. James Jan, M.D., from British Columbia's Children's Hospital in Vancouver, Canada, has effectively treated over 90 children with insomnia due to conditions such as autism, Down's syndrome, mental retardation, hyperactivity, neurological disabilities, benign sleep myoclonus (muscle spasm), certain types of epilepsy, and more. He reports in the March 1995 issue of *Developmental Medicine and Child Neurology* that no side-effects or tolerance has been found. The doses used were 2.5 mg to 10 mg, with little benefit from higher doses. Melatonin was required for two to three months, after which many of the children maintained the improved sleeping patterns without it.

Causes of Insomnia

Physical Disorders

Restless leg syndrome, gastroesophageal reflux, sleep apnea, fibromyalgia, arthritis, chronic pain, cardiac problems, congestive heart failure, emphysema, asthma, and enlarged prostate.

Psychological Difficulties

Nightmares, depression, stress, anxiety disorders, fear of insomnia, emotional discussions or arguments before bed. Chronic stress decreases the ability of pineal cells to make melatonin (Monteleone, 1993).

Improper Sleep Environment

Noise, too high or too low temperature, bed too hard or too soft, too light or too heavy blankets, snoring or restless bed partner, cats, dogs, or other pets who jump on the bed, lick your face, and want to be cuddled.

Exposure to bright light in the evening drops melatonin production within minutes. Even low level light from fluorescent lamps or light bulbs may inhibit melatonin production (Laakso, 1993).

Inadequate Sleep Habits

Too much time spent in bed reading or watching TV, daytime naps, irregular schedule.

Circadian Cycle Abnormalities

Jet lag, shift work, blindness.

Substance Overuse or Misuse

Nicotine, caffeine, alcohol, overuse of sleep medicines, amphetamine type stimulants, weight loss medicines, cold medicines such as Sudafed, herbal preparations such as ma jong which contains ephedra, and certain prescription medicines (diuretics, theophylline). Beta blockers such as Inderal (propranolol) interfere with melatonin production (Arendt, 1985); so do benzodiazepines such as Valium or Xanax. High dose corticosteroids (cortisone) in rats decreases melatonin production (Zhao, 1993).

Surprisingly, new research shows aspirin or other nonsteroidal anti-inflammatory medicines (NSAIDs) such as ibuprofen may slightly interfere with sleep (Murphy, 1994). NSAIDs suppress melatonin production.

Espresso coffee has 350 mg of caffeine per 5 oz, while drip type coffee has 140 mg. A caffeinated soft drink has 30 to 50 mg of caffeine. Tea has 20 to 50 mg, depending on how long the tea bag is brewed. An ounce of milk chocolate has 6 mg.

Alcohol induces sleep for the first few hours but the last half of the sleep cycle is interrupted and shallower. Alcohol also inhibits melatonin production (Ekman, 1993).

Jet Lag

Symptoms of jet lag include irritability, difficulty concentrating, headache, low mood, and fatigue. The change in sleeping patterns may also contribute to temporarily lowering our immunity, making us more prone to colds and infections.

Jet lag symptoms are usually worse when traveling west to east since most people have a circadian cycle longer than 24 hours (Harma, 1993). Melatonin taken in the evening of the new time zone can provide a quick readjustment.

Should melatonin be taken a few days before a trip or on the night of arrival? In a double-blind placebo-controlled trial (Petrie, 1993), 52 members of an international cabin crew were randomly assigned to 3 groups:

The early melatonin group took 5 mg starting 3 nights prior to the flight and continued 5 nights after arrival.

The late melatonin group took placebo for 3 nights before the flight then 5 mg melatonin the night of arrival and continued for 5 nights.

The third group received placebo pills throughout the study.

The late melatonin group reported significantly less jet lag and sleep disturbance following the flight compared to placebo. The late melatonin group also showed a significantly faster recovery of energy and alertness than the early melatonin group. Surprisingly, the placebo group also did better than the early melatonin group. These findings show melatonin has potential benefits for jet lag when given on the night of arrival as opposed to starting a few nights before the trip.

What dosage of melatonin should you take? As we discussed previously, a wide range of dosages works for people. An additional factor to consider with jet lag is the hours of difference between the new time zone and the one you're used to. The larger the difference, the more melatonin may be required. For instance, a dose of 3 mg may be required if you need to sleep 3 hours earlier while a 6 hour change may require more. No definite numbers can be given that apply to everyone. One rough estimate is to take 1 mg of melatonin for every hour difference. In other words, if you travel from the West Coast to the East, and there is a 3 hour change in time, take 3 mg. If you travel from the East Coast to Europe, and you need to sleep 6 hours earlier, take 6 mg.

When is the best time to take melatonin for jet lag? For most people, roughly 1 to 3 hours before the new desired bedtime works well. You may also consider splitting the dose. For instance, if you plan to take a total of 6 mg, use 3 mg about 2 hours and 1 hour before bed.

Melatonin can also be used for red-eye flights. Tommy Turner, a 37 year old banking consultant, tells me, "I've used melatonin to prevent jet lag twice. Both times I used a 2.5 mg sublingual dose. I left Atlanta a 7:30 pm and slept on the plane for 5 hours. I arrived in London the next morning, refreshed."

Shift Work

C. Boyes, a pharmacy doctoral student in Corvallis, Oregon, writes, "I work with many people at Salem Memorial Hospital who take melatonin for shift syndrome. They love it. Many of the night shift staff use it. They take a 3 mg dose about 8 am when they get off from work and state that they begin to feel drowsy about 30 minutes later. They claim to sleep better with fewer interruptions. They wake up refreshed with no hangover. I have also seen several doctors begin to routinely order melatonin as a sleep medication for their patients. We have had no complaints from patients, no apparent side effects, and it has been effective in all of the cases so far. The only side effect I have heard of was that one night shift worker said that he had a slightly upset stomach if he didn't take the medication with food."

Folkard and colleagues examined the effect of melatonin supplements on sleep, mood and behavior in a small group of police officers working spans of 7 successive night shifts. Compared to placebo, and to no treatment, melatonin (5 mg) taken at the desired bedtime improved sleep, mood, and led to increased alertness during working hours.

Workers who switch to a night shift can improve their adaptation by exposing themselves to bright artificial light at night and shielding themselves from bright light during the day. Shielding can be accomplished by wearing dark goggles during daylight hours (Eastman, 1994).

Those who regularly change work shifts, such as police officers, hospital employees, and factory workers, are more likely to get sick. They report frequent colds, fatigue, low motivation, and stomach problems. Interpersonal relationships may be affected. When an employee has been used to working 9 am to 5 pm and has to change to an 11 pm to 7 am shift, tremendous stress is placed on the body. The circadian rhythm goes haywire. Hormones are not sure when to rise or when to fall. It may take up to 2 weeks or more to completely readjust to the new schedule. Melatonin supplements can accelerate the process of re-adjustment.

Mood

Sleep disturbance influences mood and daytime energy (Totterdell, 1994). Actually, we don't need a study to tell us this, we've all experienced these symptoms after a long, toss-and-turn night. It's hard to be motivated and get things done. Melatonin can improve daytime mood in those who do not normally get a good night's sleep.

Norman, a 55 year old professor, writes, "One thing is for sure. The quality of my sleep has improved tremendously since taking 1.25 mg of melatonin nightly. Hardly ever, almost never, do I feel sleepy in the early afternoon— and this was common before I started taking melatonin. My mood is better."

I personally notice increased energy and improved mood and alertness on the days following a great night's sleep on melatonin.

In an interesting study, a male patient who lacked melatonin was given melatonin supplements. The patient's pineal gland had been destroyed 5 years earlier in the course of treatment for a pineal tumor. The administration of melatonin 0.5 mg to 2 mg significantly improved his sleep and mood (Petterborg, 1991).

Every medicine has an ideal dosage. Too high doses of melatonin may make some people tired and depressed, especially those who are prone to depression. Leonard, from Vancouver, British Columbia, writes, "I've used melatonin and it worked quite well. I've had problems getting to sleep all my life. It usually takes me about 2 hours to fall asleep and the melatonin reduced that to around a half hour, a miracle for me. I used either 3 or 6 mg depending on what I felt I would need on a given night. I slept fine without the morning grogginess from other stuff I've used over the years. I stopped using it because I noticed that I was feeling a little depressed and I suspected the melatonin. I've suffered from serious depression when I was younger— suicide attempts, the whole deal. It went away about 10 years ago. When I stopped using melatonin I returned to my usual (somewhat sleep deprived but not depressed) self again. I think it's important to look into this possible effect of melatonin. I wonder if someone has to be predisposed to depression to be affected by melatonin like I was. This experience was enough for me to give up using melatonin without regrets despite how well it worked for my insomnia." It's possible that Leonard's melatonin dose was too high for him. Since he does not sleep well, he may benefit from some additional melatonin. Perhaps his ideal dose is 0.5 or 1 mg.

Low amounts of melatonin produced by our pineal gland lead to poor sleep, and consequently cause next-day tiredness and low mood. Too high doses may also have negative effects on mood.

Melatonin doses need also to be adapted to the seasons, to menstrual cycles, to the types of food we eat, to levels of exercise, and so on. A great many factors influence melatonin levels, sleepiness, and mood. You are the best person to figure out your ideal dose.

In addition to its effects on mood, melatonin can diminish anxiety and stress. It can influence the same brain receptors that benzodiazepines, such as Valium, use to provide relaxation (Pierrefiche, 1993). However, benzodiazepines interact negatively with brain receptors involved with memory. Melatonin does not interact with these receptors, and thus does not appear to interfere with memory and learning (Neville, 1986).

We've seen how changing the patterns of our sleep cycles through traveling and shift work can produce unpleasant consequences. Just how did these sleep cycles come about, anyway? Evolutionary secrets now revealed tell a fascinating story.

SEVEN

THE CIRCADIAN CYCLE

Practically all living organisms, from the smallest amoeba to the praying mantis to a modern human, possess internal clocks that manage a variety of natural rhythms. These internal clocks evolved in order to adapt to life on this planet.

Since the earth rotates around its axis every 24 hours, with roughly 12 hours of daylight and 12 hours of night, organisms created chemicals to help them easily adapt to light and dark. It was also necessary to adapt to the varying number of hours of daylight during different seasons. Temperature, humidity, latitude, and altitude were other environmental conditions to which life has had to adapt.

Even single-celled organisms have daily rhythms regulated by melatonin or a substance with a similar chemical configuration (Reiter, 1991). Melatonin is an extremely ancient molecule and is produced by most, if not all, living creatures in the animal kingdom. Even algae are believed to have melatonin. Melatonin is not only found in every organism, but in practically every cell (Reiter, 1994). Furthermore, it has survived evolution without any chemical modifications whatsoever.

The manufacture and release of melatonin in animals and humans is a much more intricate process than that in single-celled organisms. It involves the cooperation of the pineal gland along with other regions of the brain. But in order to understand circadian rhythms, a few words are necessary about the role of...

The Pineal Gland

When I was in college during the 1970's, the pineal gland had a low status. Much like the appendix, no important bodily function was attributed to it. In physiology class, we learned about the pancreas, the liver, and the thyroid gland, but the pineal was rarely mentioned. We were taught that the pineal is a pine nut-shaped organ located somewhere in the middle of the brain. It may have played some important evolutionary role in our distant past, but no longer.

Since then medical knowledge has made amends with the once-humble pineal. We now know that the pineal gland has extremely important functions. It influences the workings of our immune system and the secretion of hormones. The pineal gland translates environmental information, such as light or temperature, into signals that are transmitted to other parts of our brain and body. This is mainly achieved through the cyclic secretion of its major hormone, melatonin.

The pineal gland does not act alone. It is intricately connected to other regions of the brain, especially the *hypothalamus*. A small section of the hypothalamus—called the *suprachiasmatic nucleus* (SCN)—is specifically, and very importantly, involved. The circadian rhythm disappears when the SCN is surgically removed or destroyed. There is constant communication between the pineal gland, other parts of the brain and spinal cord, and the SCN. Melatonin receptors have been found on the SCN.

Throughout daylight hours, light reaching the pineal gland prevents the production of melatonin. Even very low intensity light as from an indoor fluorescent light may prevent melatonin release (Laakso, 1993). Light signals reaching the pineal inhibit the activity of the enzyme that converts serotonin to melatonin. Darkness allows melatonin production. Starting in the evening, and throughout the night, the pineal gland releases melatonin, reaching peak levels between 2 and 4 am. In the morning, exposure to light shuts off melatonin production.

You may be thinking, "If the pineal gland is somewhere in the middle of my brain, how can outdoor light possibly reach it? Isn't my skull pretty thick?"

Light *photons* enter through our pupils and stimulate rods and cones in the back of our eyes, an area called the *retina*. The energy from light photons is converted to electrical and chemical impulses which are relayed through a small bundle of nerves, called the *optic tract*, to the hypothalamus. Information from the hypothalamus is in turn relayed through several other nerve tracts to the pineal gland (Aronson, 1993).

Hibernation

Animals have a great ability to adjust to fluctuating environmental conditions— they have to, otherwise they would not survive. It is essential that animals properly time their rhythms to seasonal fluctuations. They are able to endure extreme conditions of frost, heat, and shortages of food. Due to a lack of food availability in cold winter months, many go into hibernation to save energy. The shortening of daylight hours approaching wintertime allows the pineal to make more melatonin leading to hibernation. Melatonin receptors have been found both in heart and lung tissues (Pang, 1993). A higher amount of melatonin causes heart rate and breathing to slow down.

Food restriction and cold temperatures, common in winter, are also factors that induce melatonin production. (Those who have *anorexia nervosa*, consuming very little food, have been known to have higher melatonin levels [Arendt, 1992].) However, most of the time, animals adapt to seasonal changes not because of changing temperature conditions or food availability, but due to cues from length of day. The length of day is a more accurate predictor of seasons than temperature since there may occasionally be warm days in winter or cool days in summer. Melatonin provides a hormonal signal regarding day length, or, more specifically, the length of the night. Animals with seasonal breeding patterns use this signal to regulate annual reproductive cycles (Tamarkin, 1985).

Human melatonin levels also respond to changes in the length of day throughout the seasons. The 24 hour level of melatonin rhythm from saliva was measured in people living in the city of Tromso, Norway, near the Arctic circle. It was measured in January at a day length of 2 hours, in June under continuous sunshine, and in March and September at about 12 hours of light and 12 hours of darkness. Highest melatonin values were measured in January, when the least light was present (Stokkan, 1994). Similarly, a study conducted in Fairbanks, Alaska, found high levels of melatonin to be present in the blood of residents during shortened daytime hours in the winter. The researchers speculate that high daytime levels of melatonin may cause tiredness and low energy contributing to the high incidence of depression and alcoholism in Alaska and other high latitude climates (Levine, 1994). Perhaps seasonal affective disorder may also be related to high daytime melatonin levels.

Since the pineal gland is the principal area for the production of melatonin (our intestines can also make a good amount [Lee, 1993, Huether, 1992], and the retina produces small amounts [Nowak, 1989]), scientists speculate that the size of the pineal gland may have a connection with the ability of a particular species to regulate its body temperature. Animals living in high altitudes, where it is colder, tend to have larger pineal glands than those inhabiting lower altitudes. The size of the pineal even changes throughout the seasons. A bat's pineal gland is larger in winter,

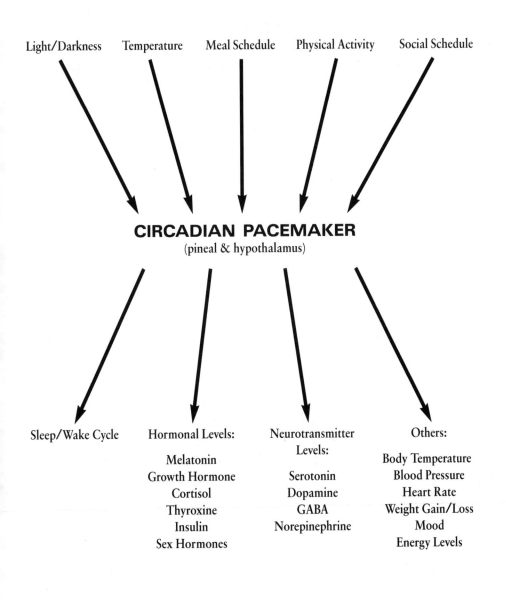

while hibernating, than in summer. When a ground squirrel had its pineal removed by surgery, it was unable to hibernate. Providing melatonin to rodents whose pineal glands are removed restores their ability to hibernate.

The light-dark cycle is the most important circadian time cue for most animals. When rodents or monkeys are kept in dim light or are experimentally blinded, their circadian rhythm becomes irregular. However, light, temperature and food restriction are not the only cues that influence circadian cycles. Humidity, perhaps, *pheromones*, and exposure to magnetic fields (Reiter, 1993) may also have an influence. It is possible that illness or infections may also modify the production and secretion of melatonin. The previous diagram summarizes both some of the influences on our circadian pacemaker and some of the effects of this pacemaker on hormones, neurotransmitter levels, and physiologic functions.

Daily Rhythms

Our hormone levels oscillate, rising and falling throughout the day, week, month, season, and year. Try this experiment. With your right index finger shut off your right nostril. Take a breath from your left nostril. Now with the same finger shut your left nostril. Take a breath from your right nostril. Most people will note that one nostril is more open than the other. Within a span of 1 to 3 hours, the open side will be closed, and the closed side will open. There is a variety of other events going on in your body at all times without your awareness. There are changes in blood sugar, blood pressure, learning ability, alertness, and mood. Even the timing of heart attacks is influenced by the time of day (Panza, 1991). There is an increased frequency of heart attacks, strokes, and sudden death during the early morning hours. This may be because platelets clump more easily and blood adrenaline levels are higher. When platelets clump they cause a clot. If this clot is in the coronary

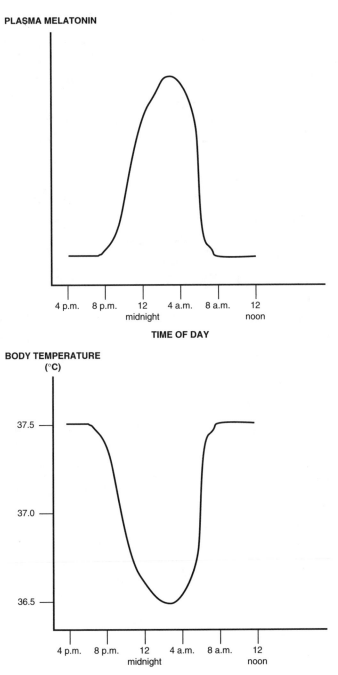

artery, a heart attack occurs. High blood adrenaline levels may induce coronary arteries to go into spasm. The circulating adrenaline levels also lead to higher blood pressure inducing the heart to pump harder and sustain more strain.

There are also daily fluctuations in body temperature, which is higher during daytime and lower at night (see Figures). There is an association between high melatonin levels and lowered nighttime body temperature (Strassman, 1991). Lower body temperatures serve to conserve calories, and thus energy. When mice are injected with a very high dose of melatonin, their body temperature drops by 2 to 3 degrees Centigrade! A study done in women showed that when they were exposed to light in the evening, shutting off melatonin production, their body temperatures rose (Cagnacci, 1993).

Now that we have become familiar with the pineal gland and the circadian rhythm, let's see how they are practically related to our bedroom, in our bed, and under the blankets.

Eight

The Science of Sleep

The earth rotates completely on its axis at 24 hour intervals. We would reasonably expect our daily sleep/wake cycle to be exactly 24 hours, too. Not so. When subjects are isolated in a chamber or cave without knowledge of night or day, a curious thing is found: they don't necessarily go to bed every 24 hours.

Aschoff, a researcher at the Max Planck institute in Germany, studied 14 human subjects in 1994. These volunteers lived singly in isolation units with no exposure to bright light and without being given cues as to time of day. Seven of the 14 were found to have a cycle of 24.5 hours. In other words, if their bedtime the first evening was at midnight, the following night it was 12:30 a.m., the next night 1 a.m., and so on. Interestingly, the remaining 7 subjects had cycles from 28 to 33 hours.

Exercise and exposure to sunlight shorten sleep cycles. In our modern society many people are deprived of direct sunshine and few engage in strenuous activities. People are exposed to indoor light at the office and again when they come home. No wonder it's a struggle to fall asleep. They probably can stay up much longer and wake up later in the morning. Keeping an active mind going late at night, by doing schoolwork, writing, or playing with the computer, adds to the problem.

There is a condition called delayed sleep phase insomnia where people develop cycles that are 26 hours or more. A person who is alert in the evenings and has difficulty falling asleep may have this long cycle— and a reflexive urge to flatten the intrusive early morning alarm clock with a hammer. A person who is sleepy in the evening and naturally wakes up early in the morning has a cycle less than 24 hours. Generally, the young have long sleep cycles which shorten as we go on in years. This accounts for the elderly going to bed earlier and waking up earlier.

In order for us to readjust a longer cycle back to 24 hours, bright light exposure is needed each day. The timing of the exposure can make a difference. When we expose ourselves to morning light, the cycle is shortened. When we expose ourselves to strong light in late evening or night, we will delay sleep and extend our cycle to more than 24.5 hours. Therefore, if you have a long cycle, and wish to shorten it, expose yourself to at least 20 minutes of outdoor light when you first wake up. If you have a short cycle, and you want to go to bed later, expose yourself to bright light in late evening.

Lessons From the Blind

Blind people have cycles similar to people who are isolated in caves or chambers (Sack, 1993). They also have a high incidence of sleep disorders. This is due to a lack of coordination between internal rhythms and the external social cues.

In a study of 20 blind people, 17 were found to have abnormal rhythms (Sack *et al.*, 1992). Many of these subjects functioned at 24 hours schedules determined by their social cues, but their biological rhythm continued at 24.5 hour cycles. They occasionally experienced insomnia and daytime sleepiness. They could tell something was not going right. The melatonin released by the brain and their sleep schedules were completely out of sync. When blind individuals are given supplemental melatonin to readjust their circadian cycle, they sleep deeper. Melatonin, when used occasionally to reset the clock, is an ideal sleep medicine for the blind.

Some blind individuals do not have completely opaque eyes. Czeisler and colleagues, from Harvard Medical School and Brigham and Women's Hospital, published the results of an interesting study in the January, 1995, issue of the *New England Journal of Medicine*. They found that even a small amount of light entering through the pupil of the eye can regulate the circadian rhythm of the blind.

Stages of Sleep

Sleep researchers have identified the following stages of sleep. (For details see *No More Sleepless Nights* by Peter Hauri, Ph.D., and Shirley Linde, Ph.D. Published by John Wiley and Sons.)

Stage

Drowsy— alpha waves

There is a drifting feeling. Eyes are closed. Muscles are relaxed. A person is still alert to the environment.

1—theta waves

There is a transition from waking to sleeping and lasts a minute to several minutes.

2— sleep spindles and K complexes

Metabolic activity decreases, blood pressure and heart rate decrease. A person can still be easily awakened and is sensitive to noise.

3 and 4— delta waves

This is called slow wave sleep. Only strong stimulation awakens people from these stages. A person is at their lowest body temperature, heart rate and blood pressure. This is restorative sleep, a time when cells repair and rejuvenate themselves. This is also the stage when sleep-talking, sleep-walking and bed-wetting are most likely to occur.

REM sleep, dream time

Rapid eye movement. Muscles are relaxed but brain waves quicken. There is increased blood flow to the brain. Blood pressure and heart rate increase, and become more variable. This stage is believed to be important for psychological health, learning, and memory consolidation.

Delta sleep, the deepest, most restorative stage, is longer in childhood, decreases at puberty, and progressively declines after age 30 (see figure). The elderly spend less time in this restorative stage and therefore are likely to feel tired in the day.

Dreaming occurs during REM sleep. Most people dream 4 or 5 times a night at about one and a half hour intervals. The first dream occurs an hour and a half after falling asleep and lasts only a few minutes. The second dream occurs about 3 hours after we sleep and lasts 10 minutes or so. Dreams progressively get longer throughout the night. The longest period of dreaming occurs in the morning before we wake up and may last up to 45 minutes.

Newborns spend almost 50% of their sleep time in REM. The percentage of REM sleep decreases to 30% by the age of 3 months and to 20% by the age of 6 months (Sandyk, 1992). Older adults spend more time in stage 1 and 2 sleep and less time in the delta stage. Waldhauser, from the University of Vienna, Austria, found in a 1990 study that melatonin administration decreases the amount of time spent in the earlier stages of sleep. Volunteers who took melatonin supplements proceeded quickly into stage 2 sleep. Deep sleep, which is stages 3 and 4, and REM sleep, lasted longer.

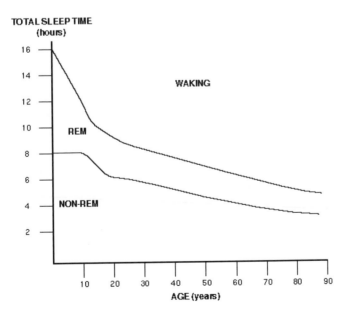

Nine

Twenty Tips for Forty Winks
how to sleep deep

1. Expose yourself to morning light by taking a walk. This tends to shorten the sleep cycle, so that when you go to bed at night, it will be easier to fall asleep. Exposure to morning sun (or very bright artificial light) will induce the pineal gland to secrete melatonin earlier in the night (Lemmer, 1994). Bright sunlight also has an energizing effect (Myers, 1993). In contrast, if you find yourself too sleepy early in the night, expose yourself to more light in late afternoon or evening (Deacon, 1994). This will tend to delay your circadian cycle so your sleep onset is postponed.

2. Exercise shortens the sleep cycle. I'm a night person; my mind is often active past midnight. However, whenever I go on an extended bicycle trip which involves riding all day long, my clock shortens to less than 24 hours. I go to bed sooner, sleep deeper, and wake up bright and early. One possible cause of insomnia in our culture is that white collar workers lead physically sedentary yet mentally active lives. When bedtime comes, the physical body is not exhausted and the mind is buzzing with thoughts— phone calls to be returned the next day, projects to be completed, etc. Contrast this to prior centuries when farmers and laborers worked in the field from dawn to dusk and were exposed to plenty of light. It's likely that they slept

very well.

Exercise can also delay sleep if performed within 3 or so hours before bedtime (Van Reeth, 1994). Melatonin secretion is delayed 1 hour if vigorous activity is done late at night (Monteleone, 1990).

3. When body temperature is raised in the late evening, it will fall at bedtime, facilitating sleep. A sauna or hot bath for at least 15 minutes serves this purpose

4. Avoid taking daily naps longer than 1 hour, or after 4 p.m., since you will be less sleepy at bedtime.

5. Caffeine in any form (sodas, chocolate, coffee, or certain teas) is best avoided after dinner. Caffeine stimulates the alertness center in the brain and can cause insomnia.

6. Consumption of alcohol in the evening may help one fall asleep, but that sleep is often fragmented and light. Alcohol inhibits melatonin secretion (Ekman, 1993). Alcohol suppresses the dream state of sleep (REM), as well as the delta phase—physiologically the deepest stage of sleep.

7. Limit late-night fluids. Liquids in the evening may prompt a middle of the night visit to the bathroom. Also, stop by the bathroom before tucking into bed.

8. Eat a small, late night snack 1 or 2 hours before bedtime. Carbohydrate meals, such as pasta or rice, stimulate insulin release which promotes the entry of blood *tryptophan* (an amino acid) into the brain. Tryptophan is converted into *serotonin* and then melatonin, inducing a calm sleep. Too large a meal before bed could, however, interfere with sleep. If you intend to eat a large meal at night, make it a few hours before bed.

In order to stay alert during the day, have some protein

included with your breakfast, such as yogurt, low-fat cottage cheese, and low-fat milk. For lunch include protein such as fish, tofu, or lean meats. If you eat a meal consisting only of carbohydrate, you will tend to become tired and sleepy.

9. Stop strenuous mental activity at least 1 hour before bedtime. Allow your mind to switch to easy reading, watching a comedy film, or television. You may also consider doing chores around the house and flossing and brushing your teeth.

10. Some people report sleeping better when taking supplements of magnesium, calcium, and B vitamins.

11. Go to bed only when you are sleepy. Use your bed only to have sex or sleep, not to watch television, eat, read, or play Nintendo.

12. If unable to fall asleep within 15 minutes, get out of bed. Don't lie there tossing and turning. Read something light, listen to the radio. Try a station you don't normally listen to. By staying in bed, your mind will associate the bed with insomnia.

13. Remove the clock from view. It only will add to your worry when constantly staring at it flashing... 2 am... 3 am... 4:30 am...

14. Unless a bedroom is completely soundproofed, many noises can disturb a deep sleep. These noises may include a dog barking; a roommate snoring; street noises such as cars, motorcycles, trucks, and police sirens; a slammed door; the refrigerator, heater or air conditioner humming; or a plane or helicopter flying overhead. Even if these noises don't awaken you, they could shift a profound, restful sleep to one that is shallow and fragmented— without your conscious realization. This is likely to interfere with daytime energy and concentration. Invest in soundproof windows or cover them with heavy drapes.

15. Use ear plugs to muffle noises. I use them every night, and sleep profoundly!

16. If light enters your bedroom in the morning, consider wearing eye shades while sleeping. Often we awaken at dawn due to sunlight slipping through the shades. This can interfere with the deepest part of our sleep.

17. Unless you are depended upon for emergencies, turn off your phone at night and turn it back on in the morning. It's a shame waking up in the middle of the night or early morning because of a wrong phone call.

18. Try a relaxation technique. There are so many to choose: progressive muscle relaxation, biofeedback, transcendental meditation, and yoga. They are all effective, you just have to find the one that works best for you. Here's a simple and quick technique that works well for many: when you are in bed, lying on your back, shake and loosen a leg and foot. Take a few slow, deep breaths by expanding your belly. Proceed to shake and loosen the other leg and foot and then return to your abdomen for a few more relaxed breaths. Proceed with this relaxation to your arms, shoulders, and neck. Now relax your facial muscles— especially the muscles around the eyes and mouth. Remember to return to your breath after relaxing each muscle group. Before you know it, you'll be drifting away.

19. Wake up at the same time each morning in order for your body to acquire a consistent sleep rhythm.

20. It's not enough to read the above tips, nod your head in approval, and say to yourself, "Great ideas." Take action! Develop your own strategies.

Ten

Melatonin and the Future

The more we learn more about this incredibly intriguing substance, the more we see its widespread influence on a variety of bodily functions. The pineal gland is involved with the hormonal system, the nervous system, and the immune system to a far greater extent than once imagined. Melatonin can also influence levels of neurotransmitters (Pozo, 1994). As a consequence of melatonin's wide influence, it has the potential to be used therapeutically in a variety of illnesses.

The following are some conditions where melatonin supplementation could be of benefit. Please keep in mind that research is still in the very early stages.

To Lower Cholesterol Levels

There is now good evidence suggesting that melatonin plays a role in various physiological functions including the metabolism of glucose, calcium and phosphorus, and the metabolism of lipids such as cholesterol and *triglycerides*. When rats have their pineal glands removed, their blood cholesterol levels become elevated. In laboratory studies, melatonin has been found to inhibit cholesterol formation (Muller-Wieland, 1994). When melatonin is given to rats with very high cholesterol levels, due either to diet or genetics, their cholesterol levels drop (Aoyama, 1988). As we get on in years, blood cholesterol levels increase. This may be due to lower melatonin levels in the elderly. Of course, cholesterol levels are affected by a number of factors, including diet, drugs, hormones, genetics, smoking and others.

To Treat Prostate Gland Enlargement

While conducting surveys for this book, I placed a question on the internet in many usenet groups, including sci.med.pharmacy and sci.life-extension. I asked people to email me any personal experiences they had using melatonin. A day later I received an email from Martin, a 56 year old accountant, who had been taking melatonin for 6 months. He wrote, "Before taking melatonin I used to get up twice a night to go to the bathroom to urinate. Now I don't get up at all, or maybe only once."

A few days later I came across information through a Medline search that melatonin is known to shrink reproductive areas including testicles, prostate, epididymis, and ovaries in rodents (Sriuilai, 1989). I thought this interesting in view of Martin's email. When the prostate gland is enlarged, it narrows the urethra, inhibiting the flow of urine. This leads to inadequate emptying of the bladder. The enlargement of the prostate gland is called benign prostatic hypertrophy (BPH). This leads men to make frequent visits to the bathroom. Frequency of urination at night is called nocturia.

To my fascination, the same night that I read the studies on melatonin's effects on the reproductive areas of rodents, I received the following email from Norman, a 55 year old professor: "I have a problem with my prostate. Nothing major, just the usual calcification and enlargement. I have not seen my urologist for the past half year, but I think the effects of the malady are less perceptible. I urinate less frequently with a much better stream. I am not willing to ascribe it to melatonin, but then again there has been no other change in my lifestyle. No question about the fact that I do not have to get up 2 or 3 times each night."

If melatonin is able to shrink the size of the prostate it could potentially have profound benefits for the millions of older men suffering from this condition. Could declining melatonin levels with age allow the prostate to grow? And will replacement melatonin shrink it back? It would be very interesting to do a study on older men with enlarged prostates and give them melatonin for 6 months to a year to see if the prostate gland shrinks and their symptoms of frequent urination improve.

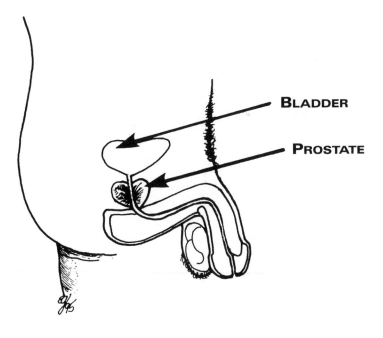

BLADDER

PROSTATE

Osteoporosis and Other Skeletal Conditions

Thinning of bones and proneness to fractures are common as we age. As discussed in Chapter 2, melatonin levels decrease as we progress in years, with postmenopausal women being especially affected. In a article published in the *International Journal of Neuroscience*, Reuven Sandyk, from Touro College in New York, surmises that the fall in melatonin levels may contribute to the development of osteoporosis. Sandyk proposes that supplementation with melatonin in post-menopausal women could be useful in preventing osteoporosis. No formal studies have yet been done. Of course, many factors besides melatonin are involved in osteoporosis, including age, diet, estrogen, smoking, physical activity, and calcium intake.

Animal research indicates that melatonin is involved in calcium and phosphorus metabolism, and other skeletal (bone) conditions as well. In an interesting study done in 1995 by Machida at the Nihon University in Tokyo, Japan, ninety chickens had their pineal glands removed on the third day after hatching. Thirty were treated with melatonin, 30 with serotonin, and the other 30 received no therapy (control group).

Scoliosis (curvature of the spine) developed in all the control group, in 22 of the serotonin group, and in only 6 of the melatonin group.

It remains to be seen how melatonin can be effectively used in the future to prevent or treat human skeletal conditions.

Cancer Treatment

In the last few years, a number of studies have assessed the role of melatonin (either acting alone or combined with other medicines) to treat or slow down the progression of cancer. The results of these studies have not reached the mainstream media.

Melatonin has been found to have a powerful inhibitory effect on some cancer cells. In tissue cultures, it has direct lethal action on estrogen-sensitive breast cancer cells (Hill, 1988; Crespo, 1994). It also inhibits prostatic carcinoma cells (Philo, 1988).

Three additional studies will be mentioned in this chapter; you can find more studies in the Reference section.

Fifty-four patients, most of them with advanced lung or colon cancer resistant to conventional therapies were given 20 mg of melatonin nightly (Lissoni, 1991). One person had a partial response, 2 had minor responses, 21 stayed stable, and the other 30 patients progressed rapidly. The researchers concluded, "These results, by showing an apparent control of the neoplastic growth and an improvement in the quality of life in a reasonable number of cancer patients for whom no other standard therapy is available, would justify further clinical trials to better define the impact of melatonin therapy on the survival and quality of life of untreatable advanced cancer patients."

Fifty patients with cancers of various forms that had metastases to the brain were split into 2 groups. The first group received supportive care (steroids and medicines to prevent seizures) while the second group received supportive care plus 20 mg of melatonin per night. The survival rate after a period of 1 year was significantly higher in those who received melatonin (Lissoni, Barni, Ardizzoia, 1994).

Forty-two patients with advanced *melanoma* and *metastases* to brain and lung received varying doses of melatonin from 5 mg a day up to 700 mg a day in 4 divided doses (Gonzalez, 1991). Advanced melanoma is a quickly progressing illness, normally fatal. After 5 weeks of treatment, 6 patients had partial responses and 6 patients had stable disease. The higher the dose, the better seemed the response. The side effects were minimal, consisting mostly of fatigue. The authors optimistically concluded "...further study of melatonin as a potentially useful agent in metastatic melanoma is warranted."

Melatonin has the potential to be used together with other medicines that treat or prevent cancer, such as tamoxifen. Human breast cancer cells in a laboratory were pre-exposed to melatonin and then exposed to tamoxifen. The pre-exposure with melatonin made the cancer cells 100 times more sensitive to the inhibitory effect of tamoxifen (Wilson, 1992).

It is also possible that, in future, people with a genetic predisposition to cancer may take nightly melatonin as a preventive measure. A study was done in mice of the C3H/Jax strain who are normally prone to develop breast tumors (Subramanian, 1991). Melatonin was given nightly from the age of 1 month to the first group. A control group did not receive any. The dose given to the mice would roughly correspond to 1-3 mg per day in humans. By the age of 1 year, 62% of the mice without melatonin had tumors, while only 23% of the mice on melatonin grew tumors.

Interestingly, blindness may have an unexpected benefit of lowering cancer rates, due to allowing more melatonin to be manufactured. No light can enter the eyes to shut off melatonin production; you may recall this being discussed in Chapter 7. There's a lower incidence of cancer in blind animals (Coleman, 1992).

Damage to DNA is hypothesized to be one of the factors involved in the beginning and progression of cancer cells. Since melatonin is an antioxidant and can protect DNA, it may slow down the rate of cancer formation.

Evidence also points to the possibility that other substances released by the pineal gland may have anti-tumor properties. An extract from the pineal gland free of melatonin was capable of inhibiting the growth of 6 types of cell lines that tend to lead to cancer (Bartsch, 1992).

Already melatonin promises to be an exciting new addition to cancer treatment. It may have a significant role to play in a variety of tumors. Lissoni and colleagues, from the division of oncological radiotherapy at Gerardo Hospital in Milan, Italy, have been on the forefront of research with melatonin in cancer. In a poster presentation published in 1994 in *Acta Neurobiologiae*, they conclude, "According to our clinical experience, melatonin has to be considered as an essential drug in the curative or palliative therapy of human neoplastic diseases."

To Treat Epilepsy

Back in 1974, Anton-Tay, an endocrinologist from Mexico City, gave six patients suffering from intractable epilepsy 2,000 mg of melatonin for 30 days as an add-on to their regular anti-seizure medicines. There was a decrease in the frequency of seizures during the treatment period.

In 1992, Golombek and colleagues, from the University of Buenos Aires in Argentina, found that giving hamsters the human equivalent dose of 3,000 mg in the early evening lowered the number of convulsions brought on by a seizure-inducing chemical known as 3-MP. Melatonin seemed to be effective by influencing the same receptors that benzodiazepines, such as Valium, influence. Benzodiazepines are known to reduce the frequency of seizures.

Although the doses of melatonin used in the above studies are very high, it is possible that much lower doses may also provide some benefits. Perhaps melatonin can be practically used in combination with other anti-seizure medicines. This approach could reduce the dose of the medicines needed for seizure control.

Schapel and fellow researchers from the Queen Elizabeth Hospital in Australia conclude their 1995 article published in *Epilepsia*, "Melatonin may have a future role in providing a more physiologic approach to treatment of the epileptics."

Improving Immunity

When aged mice with poor immunity were given melatonin, they showed improved antibody response (Caroleo, 1992). Better antibody response was associated with increased numbers of T lymphocytes and interleukin-2 production. Caroleo and colleagues conclude, "These observations suggest that melatonin may be successfully used in the therapy of immunodepressive conditions."

Please see Chapter 4 for a previous discussion on melatonin's role in immunity.

In a future printing of this book, I hope to report additional conditions that could potentially be helped by melatonin.

CAUTION

Melatonin is a very safe supplement, yet no substance is perfect. Until we know more about its long-term effects, it's best we follow the cautions listed below.

Do not use melatonin without first consulting a physician familiar with its use if:

You are pregnant.
You are breast-feeding.
You have a serious illness.
You have an *autoimmune* disorder.
You have *leukemia*, *lymphoma*, or other *lymphoproliferative* disorders.
You have a tendency for major depression.
You are presently on anti-depressants.
You are taking other medicines, especially immune suppressing medicines such as cortisol and cyclosporine.
You are diabetic or have another condition involving a hormonal imbalance.

Pregnant women or those who are considering pregnancy should definitely avoid the use of melatonin until more is known. High doses of melatonin were given to adult female rats a month before mating and throughout the whole pregnancy. The fetuses' growth was inhibited and the ovarian weight of the daughters was reduced (Diaz Lopez, 1983). This brings up the important role that melatonin plays in reproduction. Administration of melatonin normally has an inhibitory effect on sex glands, that is, it shrinks them (Ooi, 1989). When male golden hamsters are given melatonin, there is shrinking of the testicles with a decrease in the production of sperm cells (Raynaud, 1989). In animal studies melatonin has been found to inhibit testosterone production (Persengiev, 1991). Melatonin is being studied as a safe medicine for contraception (Silman, 1993). As mentioned in Chapter 1, low doses of melatonin, 2 mg, given to humans nightly for 2 months, did not effect testosterone or other hormone levels (Terzolo, 1990). Melatonin's inhibitory effects on gonads is likely to be minimal or none at low doses.

Melatonin is known to go through breast milk and thus is likely to pass to a nursing baby. It's possible that high levels of melatonin reaching a baby may lead to sleepiness and lethargy.

Since melatonin improves and stimulates the immune system, it could possibly have detrimental effects in conditions where the immune system is already out of control. These include autoimmune diseases such as systemic lupus erythematosus (SLE), or lymphoproliferative conditions such as leukemias and lymphomas. Persengiev (1993) reports melatonin administration in vitro (in test tube) caused an increase in *myeloma* cell proliferation. No conclusive clinical studies of the effect of melatonin on the above illnesses have been published; therefore, consult a physician before using melatonin if you suffer from any of these conditions.

What about taking melatonin concurrently with other medicines? No formal clinical research is available on this issue. There are many medicines, and an infinite number of potential combinations. It would be almost impossible to test melatonin with each one. It is best at this point not to initiate melatonin use if you're already regularly using other medicines until we know more. This certainly applies to anti-depressants such as *monoamine oxidase inhibitors* and *serotonin reuptake inhibitors*.

John, a businessman and frequent traveler, writes, "I have used melatonin a number of times to reset my body clock on business trips (I live out west and travel east). Taking 3-6 mg a couple of hours prior to local midnight does the trick. One little problem... the last time I did this, I think I took 6 or 9 mg, I woke up about 2 am with a panic attack. I have experienced anxiety before, but nothing like this. It was all I could do to keep from running screaming out of the motel room. It was a feeling of total immediate fear, with nothing at all to be afraid of— real or imagined. A very odd experience to be scared to death, but not afraid of anything! After about 10 minutes of sitting there panicked and afraid to move, I dug out some Xanax, took it, and about 20 minutes later, after the Xanax started to work, I was able to get back to sleep.

"At the time, I was taking Paxil [a Prozac relative] for depression, so this may be some sort of interaction. Since then, needless to say, I have been afraid to take melatonin. I don't know if anyone else has ever reported this effect, but it was probably a result of melatonin (possibly combined with the Paxil). I have never had this experience before or since."

Paxil and other selective serotonin reuptake inhibitors are suspected to increase the melatonin amplitude at night (Skene, 1994). Whether this had anything to do with John's panic attack is unclear at this time. Monoamine oxidase inhibitors also increase melatonin levels (Oxenkrug, 1988).

Since melatonin enhances the immune system, it may counteract the effects of immune suppressing medicines. Melatonin also influences various hormonal levels when given in high doses; therefore, diabetics, people with thyroid problems, those with adrenal disorders, etc., should consult a physician before initiating use.

Side effects with melatonin use that have thus far been reported in my surveys of over 200 people include:

Grogginess or 'fuzzy thinking' in the morning— 15%.
Worse sleep than normal— 5%.
Bad dreams or nightmares— 5%.
Waking up in the middle of the night with a low mood— 2%.
Mild headache— 2%.
Low sex drive with chronic use— 2%.
Depressed feelings with chronic use— 2%.
Mild stomach upset with pills— 1%.

Please note that more varieties of side effects may be reported in the future as more and more people use melatonin. Side effects are minimal or none with doses less than 1 mg. Most of the above side effects have been infrequent and were reported by people taking more than 3 mg. All disappeared upon discontinuation. Another factor to consider is that side effects are reported by research subjects even when they are given placeboes.

Joe Kraska, a software developer from Vista, CA, provides us with an account of a bad experience. He writes, "I am a 27 year old male and find melatonin to be the most effective sleeping aid that I've ever tried. The only bad effect I ever had from melatonin was when I first started. Day 1, I used 2.5 mg and liked the result. Day 2, I tried 5 mg to see what would happen. I awoke in the middle of the night with a crushing depression, and felt like I was going to cry. I could not sleep. Afterwards, I laid off for a couple of days, and then went back to 2.5 mg. After several weeks, I tried 5 mg again— with no negative results.

"Users should treat melatonin like a drug, cautiously and seriously. It clearly affects human neurotransmitter biology. I tell all my friends that they should start off with small doses and work their way up to what works for them without going overboard."

What about the purity of melatonin?

There are a great number of melatonin manufacturers and retailers. Since melatonin is not regulated by the FDA, its purity cannot be guaranteed. This is also true of many supplements, medicines, vitamins, and herbal products bought over the counter.

My hope, and that of many others, is that as the popularity of melatonin increases, wholesalers and manufacturers will take advantage of independent testing companies that analyze and certify the purity of melatonin batches. This certification would ease the concerns of many who wish to use melatonin regularly but are worried about possible impurities.

The Chemistry of Melatonin

Melatonin is made from an *amino acid* called *tryptophan*. Tryptophan is an essential amino acid, that is, the body cannot make it; we need to get it from the foods we eat. Tryptophan is found in a wide variety of foods. As we consume tryptophan during the day, the body converts it into *serotonin*, an important brain chemical involved with mood. Serotonin, in turn, is converted into melatonin (see figure). This conversion occurs most efficiently at night.

The chemical name of melatonin is N-acetyl-5-methoxy-tryptamine. It is made naturally in the pineal gland, the retina, and the intestines. It's possible that larger amounts than previously thought may be formed in the intestines.

In the pineal gland, tryptophan is converted to serotonin by 5-hydroxylation and decarboxylation. An acetyl group is added to serotonin by an enzyme called serotonin-N-acetyl-transferase (NAT). NAT is believed to be the rate limiting enzyme, that is, the amount of melatonin produced depends on the activity of this enzyme. Activation of NAT depends not only on signals induced by light hitting the retina, but from information relayed from other parts of the brain. Vitamin B6 is involved in aiding NAT. You will often find B6 added to melatonin pills or lozenges. The rationale for this is not clear to me since, by providing preformed melatonin, there would be no need for the additional B6.

The acetylation of serotonin is followed by adding a methyl

group, leading to the molecule of this book, melatonin. When rats and chicks are given a large dose of tryptophan, melatonin levels in the blood rise (Huether, 1992). This is probably why taking tryptophan induces sleepiness.

A few years ago tryptophan was available as a supplement over the counter. Unfortunately, a batch from Japan was contaminated with a toxin which caused a disease called eosinophilia-myalgia syndrome. Over a thousand people became ill with a few dying. The FDA took tryptophan off the market as a cautionary measure until more information became available. It is now known for certain that tryptophan was not the cause of the illness, the toxin was. Tryptophan has not been available to the American consumer since it was taken off the shelves.

Melatonin is metabolized to very interesting compounds, including 5-methoxy-tryptamine. This chemical may be involved in inducing REM sleep with vivid dreams. 5-methoxy-tryptamine is further metabolized to N,N-dimethyl-5-methoxy-tryptamine and other tryptamines. Our brain manufactures its own hallucinogens, which lead us to dream. I can envision headlines in the news someday, "FDA declares dreaming illegal!"

For full details about melatonin's metabolism, see the references mentioned in Chapter 3.

Opposite page: Metabolism of tryptophan, serotonin, and melatonin.

NAT is N-acetyl-transferase

HIOMT is hydroxyindole O-methyl-transferase

AAA is aryl acylamidase

OH is hydroxyl, CH_3O is methoxy, COOH is carboxyl, and CH_3CO is acetyl.

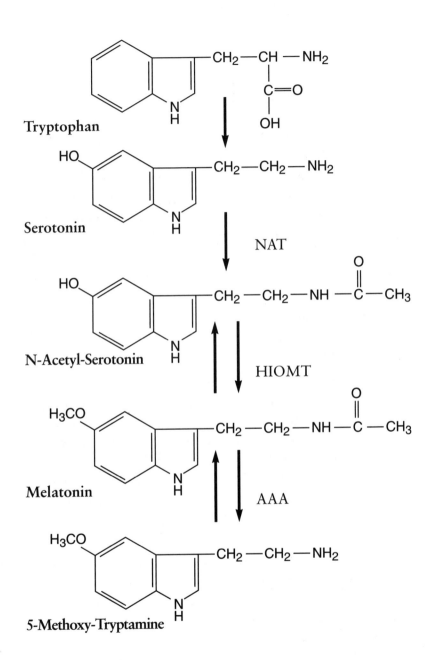

Tryptophan

Serotonin

NAT

N-Acetyl-Serotonin

HIOMT

Melatonin

AAA

5-Methoxy-Tryptamine

Frequently Asked Questions (FAQ)

Will I get darker or lighter if I take melatonin?

Many people confuse the word melatonin with the skin pigment melanin. They are different compounds although studies have shown that melatonin can influence coat color in animals and skin color in amphibians. McElhinney and colleagues wanted to investigate the effect of melatonin on human skin color. They followed seven patients receiving orally administered melatonin over a mean duration of 19 months. There was no significant change in skin color among patients receiving melatonin. Nordlund and Lerner gave 1000 mg of melatonin for one month to 5 individuals with hyperpigmented skin due to metabolic abnormalities. Melatonin lightened the hyperpigmented skin of one patient with untreated adrenogenital syndrome, but had no effect on the other four. Incidentally, this high dose did not induce any toxicity. All blood tests, eye exams, blood pressure, pulse, urine test, etc. were normal. The only side effect reported was drowsiness.

Does diet influence melatonin production?

A carbohydrate meal such as pasta, grains, legumes, fruit juices, etc., elevates blood sugar levels which triggers the pancreas to release insulin. Insulin allows blood sugar (glucose) to enter cells and thus lowers glucose levels in the bloodstream. Insulin also allows an amino acid in the blood called tryptophan to enter the brain more easily. Tryptophan is then converted to serotonin which is, in turn, converted to melatonin. Therefore, a small to moderate meal of carbohydrates (preferably complex) in the evening an hour or two before bed can promote sleep.

An interesting study in rats showed that, in the long run, a diet with adequate amounts of fish oils or polyunsaturated fatty acids such as in safflower oil allowed the pineal gland to be more responsive to making melatonin than a diet deficient in these fatty acids (Gazzah, 1993).

I've been taking a pharmaceutical sleep medicine for the past eight months. Is it possible that I could switch to melatonin?

Use of most pharmaceutical medicines results in tolerance. They lose some of their effectiveness with time. Furthermore, there are withdrawal symptoms such as insomnia for up to a month or more after stopping them. Discuss with your physician on how you can slowly taper your dose over a period of weeks. Follow the twenty tips as outlined in chapter eight. Introduce melatonin slowly in low doses as you taper off the pharmaceutical sleeping pill. There have not been any studies yet on the effectiveness of melatonin in those who are used to strong sleeping pills. It's possible high doses of melatonin, up to 10 mg, may be required. It's also possible you may be able to reduce your dose of a sleeping pill when you take it along with melatonin.

A few years ago tryptophan, an amino acid and sleep medicine, was contaminated with a toxic agent and some people died. Could this happen with melatonin?

Contamination can happen to any substance whether it be a pill, food, water, air, etc. Melatonin supplements are not any more, or less, likely to get contaminated than any other product that we ingest. Furthermore, it is not fair to compare a contamination of a sleep medicine such as tryptophan to possible contamination with melatonin.

Both aspirin and acetaminophen (Tylenol) lower fever. Using the above illogical argument one could argue that since Tylenol products were laced with cyanide a few years ago and seven people died, then aspirin products are likelier to also get laced.

I'm diagnosed with narcolepsy. Is melatonin helpful with this condition?

Narcolepsy is characterized by a sudden uncontrollable disposition to sleep. This occurs at irregular intervals throughout the day, with or without an obvious predisposing cause. It can be very dangerous, especially when driving on the freeway or operating heavy machinery. The cause is likely due to a disturbed circadian sleep/wake cycle. Some cases similar to narcolepsy occur when the pineal gland is surgically removed. High doses of nightly melatonin, up to 50 mg, have shown some benefit in patients suffering from narcolepsy. Scheduled naps, daytime use of stimulants, and small, frequent meals that include protein are some other methods of treatment. You may also try a portion of a 500 mg tyrosine or phenylalanine capsule (available in health food stores) early in the morning. These amino acids will help you stay alert. Consult your physician before taking these amino acids since in some people they can increase blood pressure. People who are phenylketonurics of course should not take phenylalanine.

I suffer from seasonal affective disorder (SAD). Would taking melatonin help?

Seasonal changes in mood and energy have long been accepted as part of life in the far north (Booker, 1992). Interestingly, those who are newcomers to a northern country are affected by winter blues much more than natives who have been living in that environment for generations. For instance, native Icelanders whose families have been living in Iceland for centuries suffer SAD at a much lesser rate than individuals who have recently migrated. Could the genetic code somehow adapt to an environment's seasonal changes and this information be passed on to progeny?

Most of the symptoms of SAD begin during the fall when daylight becomes progressively shorter. These symptoms include irritability, fatigue, low mood, weight gain, and carbohydrate craving. There is an increase in the number of hours spent in bed from an average of seven to nine. SAD is four times as common in women as in men. Exposure to bright artificial light improves many of these symptoms. Physical activity, such as jogging, also helps.

Depressive symptoms last longer the farther north one lives. As many as 90% of people living above a latitude of 40 degrees north may experience seasonal changes in mood and behavior, and about one fourth of them consider these changes to be a problem (Harris, 1993). Oregon in the West, Nebraska in the midwest, and Pennsylvania in the East are states that are located above the 40 degree latitude.

A study conducted in Fairbanks, Alaska, found high levels of melatonin to be present in the blood of residents during daytime hours in the winter. The researchers speculate that high daytime levels of melatonin may cause tiredness and low energy accounting for the high incidence of depression and alcoholism in Alaska and other high latitude climates (Levine, 1994).

A recent study (Schlager, 1994) published in the *American Journal of Psychiatry* reports an interesting finding. When patients with winter depression are given propranolol (Inderal), a beta blocker normally used for high blood pressure or heart disease, they got better. Beta blockers stop melatonin production. The timing of the dosage is critical. The researchers found a dosage of 40 mg of propranolol in the early morning, at about 5:30 am, provided improvement in the majority of patients.

In two studies, treatment of SAD patients with melatonin has not been found to be effective (Wirz-Justice, 1990), and even made symptoms worse (Rosenthal, 1986). Even though research studies have not found melatonin therapy to be effective, I have received notes from survey respondents who find it helpful. Mary, 28 years old, says, "I have noticed that regularly taking melatonin in the winter months seems to help me avoid depression caused by shorter day length. I usually take one 3 mg tablet one hour before bedtime." Elaine, another respondent, writes, "Since reading an article on the use of small doses of melatonin to induce sleep and reading speculation about its possible effect on seasonal affective disorder, I have used melatonin this fall and winter to sleep. For me, one of the symptoms of SAD is insomnia. I find melatonin to be amazingly effective, without any apparent side effects."

As you can see, there are conflicting reports on the benefits of melatonin supplements in SAD. Perhaps the answer may lie in having adequate amounts of melatonin at night and to find ways to shut off melatonin production during the day. During the winter, a shorter day length allows more melatonin to be produced during the day which can lead to tiredness (Danilenko, 1994). Perhaps the reserves of serotonin are converted to melatonin and a shortage of serotonin leads to low mood.

The nightly peak of melatonin production is less in the winter, with a phase delay. This phase delay would mean that SAD patients will tend to be sleepier later in the evening. One possible treatment approach for SAD could be to provide a small dose of melatonin at night as a supplement to induce restful sleep and advance the phase delay, and then shut off production in the morning by light therapy or treatment with a beta blocker. This approach would allow high levels of melatonin at night and very little or none during the day.

Personal Stories of Melatonin Users

"I take melatonin solely for anti-aging purposes and have done so for 2 years. The first year I took 6 mg and this year I increased it to 9 mg. I fall asleep quicker and sleep sounder. Dreams are slightly more intense. I have not noticed any other side effects."

Larry, 53, CA

"I have had positive effects, feeling more refreshed in the morning, my menstrual periods are much lighter and not as uncomfortable. My dosage has been 3 mg per night. It seems remarkable as far as the sleeping goes. That puffy eyed feeling that you've really been in deep sleep, I haven't experienced in many years until taking melatonin.

"The negative effect that I am most concerned and perplexed about is that I appear to have become much more anti-social than ever before. I've always been a bit of hermit but now, any socializing is dreaded. Once socializing, I usually enjoy it but it doesn't seem to help me look forward to the next social experience. I mainly want to have a lot of privacy and enjoy my many hobbies and interests such as reading, gardening, and playing with my dog. I am married and my relationship seems to be OK, but my husband isn't very happy with my lack of sociability.

"I have also noticed my being much less willing to confront when necessary. I've always been somewhat on the aggressive side; always standing up for myself. Now I seem to back down easily. I overpaid a local M.D., for example, $300.00, but instead of going thru the work to try to get it back, I just decided to let it go.

"Some of my symptoms could be pre-menopausal psychological changes. Perhaps I'm suffering from some type of depression brought on by menopause?

"I'm giving melatonin, 10 mg, to my dog and it has helped considerably in my efforts to get him off of steroids (prednisone) due to allergies and skin problems."

AA, age 49

"I took half a 3 mg tablet and had a trippy nightmare of people melting into the mud. This seemed kind of appropriate to the fact that I was sleeping in Moscow and Russia is backsliding."

Bill R

"Several years ago I was diagnosed with sleep apnea after sleep studies were done because of daytime fatigue and an observation by my wife that I seemed to stop breathing at times during the night. Most of the pharmaceutical sleeping pills are not recommended for this condition so I have been looking for some natural means of falling asleep since I do have periodic insomnia. I came across some mention of melatonin in a lay magazine and decided to try it. It worked too well in the usual 3 mg dose. I was drowsy most of the next day and I also had trouble waking up. I began cutting the dose down till I now take about 1 mg at times and often just 0.5 mg. I have been using it for 3 months now taken 30 minutes before bedtime.

"I have suggested melatonin to several friends and they took it with little effectiveness because they were used to taking Dalmane, Restoril, or Xanax. One of these individuals tried it once in a 3 mg dose and said that it made him feel depressed the next day."

Sam, 71, retired family physician, CA.

"Before I came across melatonin, it felt as if all my biological cycles were going out of sync. I would lie in bed, become 'asleep', but not benefit from it. I had given myself another three to six months before I became totally non-functional.

"Then I tried staying up one whole cycle a week. Friday night, I would not go to bed, and aside from one short nap, not sleep till Saturday night. This would work, but would wear off by Thursday.

"After multiple attempts at trying 'blinking lights' treatments and theta rate entrainment, finally someone told me about melatonin. AH! MELATONIN. I took two, but it failed to make me drowsy. When I did go to sleep, I fell asleep, and slept well. Yes, upping the dose would make me drowsy the next day, but that felt A LOT better than the frazzled feeling I had had before melatonin!

"In the beginning, I would alternate between two 3 mg pills a night and three 3 mg pills a night. As the months passed, I needed less and less. By six months I could skip a night. Now, I may take it once or twice a week, whenever I remember."

John, 44, San Francisco, CA

"I have been taking 3 mg of melatonin for nearly two years. I sleep a good 7 hours and wake up feeling well rested. I can skip taking it with no problems. The cycle seems well established. I have no unusual side effects. Dreaming is about the same as it ever was. The studies that indicate potential of melatonin to prevent some forms of cancer are encouraging enough to me to continue with it."

Al, 50, Philadelphia, PA

"I have been taking 2.5 mg of melatonin at night for a couple of months now. It seems to promote a refreshing sleep, with vivid dreams. I now sleep a complete 6 hours instead of shallow 8 hours.

"No objective reason for this opinion except how I feel, and I may be wrong in attributing this to melatonin, but I think it creates a sense of slightly unnatural calm (tranquilizer effect) and, more noticeably, mild depression. The slight misery does not really seem to have an objective cause and it's much more an emotion than a thought process. As I have a high level of internal happiness, I think the melatonin may be responsible for mild depression. It may depress libido too."

Iain, 37, Los Angeles

"I am a research physician at the Naval Health Research Center. I take melatonin to get to sleep and to reset my sleep/wake cycle. I do this usually Sunday night because I am a night person and have to get up at 5:30 am on Monday morning. It works wonders. I had no idea what to expect while taking it so I had no preconceived expectations. I noticed that I seemed to have vivid dreams on those nights. They always seemed to be significant and related to some problem I had been concerned with. This does not surprise me because dreams come from the unconscious mind. It seems that the melatonin makes it easier for the unconscious to surface in the form of dreams. Now I take it if there is something bothering me and I can't figure it out. I take 10 mg 2 hours before I want to sleep."

Lisa

"I've had problems with my intestines for over 10 years. I saw a number of doctors and they diagnosed me as having irritable bowel syndrome. Basically, I wake up at 3 am with bloating and gas, and have to go to the bathroom. This disrupts my sleep. For some reason, the symptoms don't happen as much during the day. I tried various diets with no help. A physician said I should go on a relaxing pill at night such as Elavil. I didn't want to take a medicine like that.

"One day, as I was walking through my local drugstore, I noticed a bottle of melatonin. I had never heard of it before but it said on the bottle that it was natural and it was used for sleep. I took a 3 mg pill that night. It was amazing. I did not get up at all during the night. It's been 3 months that I've been taking it and it's worked wonders. I can't believe it!

"I haven't noticed any tolerance. My dreams seem to be more complicated with more intricately interwoven plots."

Lansing Holmes, 71, LCSW, Brentwood, CA

"I just started using melatonin at 3 mg one hour before bedtime and have noticed my dreams to be very vivid and detailed, and altogether pleasant, so far.

"I can also attest to the fact that the melatonin has greatly enhanced my ability to fall asleep quickly. Although I still seem to wake up at least once during the night, I have no trouble in relaxing and falling back asleep in just a few minutes. I feel very rested by my usual rising time."

Casey emailed again two weeks later.

"I and my significant other have both observed that my general mood for the last couple of weeks has been more cheerful than usual. I'm not a particularly dour person by nature or anything, but I definitely feel a more positive attitude towards life, which I attribute to at least being able to have consistently restful nights.

"I have noticed that the vivid dreaming I experienced the first week I started taking melatonin seems to have subsided."

Casey Bahr, 40, Hillsboro, OR

"I used melatonin for the first time last night. A 2.5 mg sublingual tablet. Soon after taking it I felt a little sleepy, but it took me longer than usual to go to sleep. I woke up at some unknown time during the night, and then woke up at 5:30 am. I lay in bed half asleep until my usual wake-up time, during which time I had a pleasant dream."

Brian

"I've had severe chronic insomnia and I've tried using melatonin. The first time I used it, I thought I was asleep and dreaming, then I sat up in bed and opened my eyes and looked around and realized I was awake, yet somehow the dream kept going in my head. I later fell asleep and dreamt normally, so I don't remember what the dream was about.

"I did try melatonin again last weekend. On Friday night I took 9 mg at about 4 am. It did seem to help me sleep. I tried it again on Sunday, and that time it felt like it made 'bursts' of some kind (don't know how else to describe it), and I couldn't fall asleep at all that night. I thought this was also an unpleasant experience, so I don't think I'll try melatonin again.

"I know I've probably got the weirdest reaction."

Wayne, 24, computer programmer, Seattle, Washington

"I'm a 26 year old computer programmer and have used melatonin approximately 6 times for sleep. I stopped taking them about a year ago because I could not find a dose low enough to put me to sleep without making me really groggy the next day. Usually within 15-20 minutes after taking it (1mg or less) I would be yawning VERY hard and have to sleep within the next 5 minutes or so. The next morning I would sleep longer than usual if not for my trusty alarm clock.

"I gave the rest of the bottle to a 39 year old friend from work. He is normally a very agitated person and will stay up working on projects till 4 am because he can't fall asleep. Because of this, he uses Xanax. He was complaining about not being able to sleep during the time he was trying to drag himself off reliance on Xanax. He loved the melatonin."

Rodney Reid, Milwaukee, WI

"I use it occasionally to improve sleep, and it seems to work pretty well. I do notice vivid dreams when I use melatonin— which I like. I use sublingual lozenges. My mother claimed that melatonin had no effect on her at all. On a recent visit, I saw she was using melatonin pills made from pineal extract. I gave her a lozenge from another company with melatonin made synthetically. She noticed a pronounced effect. She tried it for a short time and then had an aggravation of a chronic reproductive system infection (she's had it for >20 years) that she thinks is hormone dependent. This infection flares up not infrequently, so it isn't clear if there was a cause-effect relation."

Steve Dunn, 38, computer programmer, Boulder, CO

"I definitely have noticed more energy in the day. My mood is better and I don't get the urge to nap in the day as I used to. Before melatonin I would have an irresistible urge to snooze in the afternoon. This would mess up my whole sleep cycle since that night I wouldn't be able to fall asleep at a reasonable time. I would stay up late, and feel lousy the next day. Melatonin has been a godsend.

"It's been 5 months that I've been taking melatonin, a third of a 2.5 lozenge, about 4 or 5 times a week. I take it an hour before bed. No side effects, occasional vivid dreams. I wish researchers would do some long-term studies in humans to see if it's safe to use forever."

Regina, 56, librarian, Miami, Florida

"I have been using melatonin for about six weeks now and have very good experiences with it. I used to wake up what literally felt like hundreds of times a night and was often tired. I haven't noticed any harmful side effects and my sleep has improved even when I'm not taking it (like on weekends)."

CF, 23, Alaska

"The first night I took one 3 mg tablet and had a horrible sleep with nightmares. Since I have had experience with Effexor (an antidepressant) that some of the medications for fibromyalgia make you feel worse when you start taking them, I persevered. The next 7 nights I felt that my sleep had improved somewhat. I still woke up at night 4 or 5 times, but when I slept, it was in a deeper sleep. I then called my internist and asked him whether I could increase the dosage; he approved. I have now been taking 2 tablets per night. I have improved a little more; now I only wake up 2 or 3 times during the night, and sleep is more restful, but I still wake up in the morning feeling like I have not had enough rest. The last few days I have also awakened with a backache; I am not sure whether this is a result of the fibromyalgia trigger points flaring up or if it is connected to the melatonin.

"I am debating whether to go to 3 tablets per night. I really need to get more rest at night since I have a full-time job and family responsibilities. Right now, I work all week just waiting for the weekend when I can sleep a little later or take a nap in the middle of the day...Unfortunately, I can't always do either."

CB, Upton, NY

"I have used melatonin at 1.25 mg for six weeks 30 minutes before bedtime. I haven't had lucid dreams and no morning drowsiness. When I use 3 mg, I notice drowsiness in the morning."

AW, London, England

"My wife, 39 years old, has been taking 3 mg of melatonin prior to bed for the past 3 or 4 months. She has developed mild facial hair and is concerned that the melatonin has caused it."

David

"I take melatonin 3 mg just before bedtime for fibromyalgia type problems and it works better than anything my doctor has come up with over the past 15 years. If I skip the melatonin one night, I can definitely tell the next morning with more muscle pain and lower energy. Melatonin is the ONLY sleep enhancer that I have tried that doesn't leave me groggy and 'hung over' the next morning. I wake up fairly early, with a clear mind, and it is much easier to get out of bed than with any other medication that I have taken."

Roger

"After the January, 1994 Los Angeles earthquake I had difficulty sleeping. The quake shook me up real bad. I tossed and turned in bed for weeks, constantly worried about being shaken again. I was becoming a nervous wreck. I couldn't think clearly at work. A friend suggested melatonin. I took 3 mg for five nights. It helped me tremendously get over my fear of sleeping again. It's now been over a year and I haven't felt the need to take it since then."

Carol, 24, Sherman Oaks, CA

"I've used melatonin a few times now and find my sleep is quite deep and my dreams are vivid. I haven't noticed any side effects."

Robert Butterworth, Ph.D., clinical psychologist, Los Angeles

"I took half of a 5 mg lozenge during the day because I was under a lot of stress and hadn't slept well for 2 nights. I fell asleep very fast, and my dream was quite unusual. I saw a little man the size of a thumb in a black suit and tie who told me, 'You don't need me anymore, I'm leaving you.' With those words I woke up and felt so great, as if something really heavy had lifted off my shoulders. It was a wonderful and healing experience."

Yelena Malysheva, teacher, Los Angeles

"I was prescribed doxepin for partial chronic fatigue, allergies, and insomnia. It helped a great deal and I took it for a year. During that time, I also experimented with melatonin when I had periods of severe insomnia and doxepin didn't help. As long as I kept the melatonin dose at half of a 2.5 mg sublingual lozenge, it provided a fairly dramatic improvement in sleep, mood, and late-day energy.

"After a year, I also added Prozac in an attempt to further improve my late-day energy level. Prozac worked wonders. However, the effect of melatonin while taking Prozac is less significant. It will help me fall asleep very quickly, but there appears to be an increased tendency to wake up earlier than normal, presumably from downregulation of the melatonin receptors."

Scott Newman, Ph.D., Western State College, Gunnison, CO

"I am still trying different dosages, ranging from 6-12 mg before bed, then 6 mg when I wake up early (which is my problem). I have had no change in dreams. The reason I am waking up early is that I am taking a central nervous system stimulant, pemoline (Cylert), for the afternoon fatigue caused by my *multiple sclerosis*. I have noticed no side effects, but am very concerned about the possibility of such (although it does seem to me that melatonin ought to be safe). My neurologist has never heard of melatonin (!) but did call the manufacturers, who claimed there was no interaction with pemoline."

SB, 49, New Haven, Connecticut

"I have taken about 300 doses of 3 mg pills over the last year. My dreams have not changed, but my mood has improved, I have more energy, and my sex drive may be better. There has been no tolerance and no physical addiction. Perhaps it is habit forming since I took melatonin frequently to help me get a deeper sleep. I stopped using it after a year since I learned some mental relaxation techniques to sleep better. There were no withdrawal symptoms. I still use it when I travel to regulate time zone shifts."

Bruce Brown, Private Investigator; author of The Cheap Date Handbook

"I have taken 3 mg just before bedtime on perhaps 15-17 occasions. I have the sensation that I usually have a deeper night's sleep whenever I take it, but I frequently wake up with a groggy, almost hungover feeling, as if I had slept too long (even when I've only slept my usual amount)."

EP, Chicago, Illinois

"I took Zoloft [a Prozac relative] for half a year to improve my mood and reduce daytime fatigue. It was moderately effective. Then, four months ago, I added melatonin, a 3 mg capsule nightly. I found I slept better and more easily, although not longer. I also discovered my mood improved significantly, and have now stopped taking Zoloft. This makes me wonder if some people who think they are depressed are simply not sleeping well.

"One of my two dogs died recently from cancer. The other, a Doberman-Shepherd-Retriever mix, acted sad and snapped at people until I started sprinkling 1 mg of melatonin on his food each night. Now he is calmer and friendlier, and even barks less."

Russell Kurtz, Ph.D., Culver City, CA

Glossary

Alzheimer's disease— a progressive brain disease leading to memory loss, interference with thinking abilities, and other losses of mental powers. Brain cells show degenerative damage.

Amino acid— a molecule that serves as a unit of structure of proteins. It contains nitrogen. Twenty-two amino acids are found in the human body, such as arginine, lysine, tryptophan, and phenylalanine. Eight of these are essential, that is, the body cannot make them. They need to be ingested through foods.

Anorexia nervosa— a condition, mostly in women, characterized by abnormal body image, extremely low food consumption, thinness, and sometimes leading to death from starvation.

Antibody— a protein molecule made by white blood cells that combines with bacteria, viruses, and toxins to neutralize them.

Antigen— a substance or toxin to which the body reacts by forming antibodies.

Antioxidant— a substance that combines with damaging molecules, neutralizes them, and thus prevents the deterioration of DNA, lipids, and proteins. ß-Carotene and vitamins C and E are the best known antioxidants, but more and more are being discovered each year. It is believed that one aspect of aging is the slow degeneration and breakdown of chemicals within our cells. Antioxidants prevent or slow down this degenerative process. Melatonin is a powerful antioxidant.

Autoimmune— immunity against self. The body makes antibodies that attack and damage its own cells. Systemic lupus erythematosus is one such condition.

Cell membrane— a thin layer consisting mostly of fatty acids that surrounds each cell.

Chromatin— the genetic material of a cell's nucleus, including DNA.

Circadian— body rhythms associated with the 24 hour cycle of the earth's rotation. There are changes in blood pressure, blood sugar, mood, energy level, arousal, and hormone levels.

Cortisol (hydrocortisone)— a substance secreted by the adrenal glands (located above the kidneys). It is a steroid. High doses lead to interference with the proper functioning of the immune system.

Emphysema— a lung disease involving damage and destruction to alveoli (lung cells). Smoking is one of the most common causes.

Eosinophil— a type of white blood cell that greatly increases in number in certain allergic diseases or when the immune system is trying to fight an infection by a parasite. It also has the ability to form chemicals, such as interleukin 2, that fight cancer.

Gonad— a testicle or ovary.

Hypothalamus— a small area of the brain above and behind the roof of the mouth. The hypothalamus is prominently involved with the functions of the autonomic nervous system and the hormonal system. It also plays a role in mood and motivation.

Immune Globulins— a group of proteins found in blood. Immune globlins (or immunoglobulins) fight off infections by attaching to and killing bacteria and viruses. The best known is gamma globulin.

Interferon— a small protein produced by white blood cells to fight infections, especially viral, and some forms of cancer.

Interleukin— similar to interferon, a small protein produced by white blood cells to fight infections and some forms of cancer. There are many types of interleukins, numbered 1, 2, 3, etc.

Leukemia— a form of cancer that results in the abnormal production of white blood cells. It can be a slow onset, called chronic, or a sudden onset, called acute.

Lou Gehrig's disease— also known as amyotrophic lateral sclerosis, it is a degenerative disease of the nerve cells that control muscular movement. Recently it has been found that a genetic shortage of an antioxidant enzyme, called superoxide dismutase, may lead to the progression of this disease.

Lymphocyte— a type of white blood cell. Those made in the *b*one marrow are called B lymphocytes while those made in the *t*hymus gland are called T lymphocytes.

Lymphoma— any of a group of diseases characterized by painless, progressive enlargement of lymph glands. Hodgkin's disease is a form of lymphoma.

Lymphoproliferative— any condition that involves uncontrolled growth and multiplication of immune cells.

Macrophage— a type of white blood cell that ingests and destroys other cells, bacteria, viruses, or foreign matter in the blood and tissues.

Melanin— a dark brown or black pigment that normally occurs in skin and hair. It is formed by oxidation of tyrosine or tryptophan to dopamine and further oxidation to melanin.

Melanoma— a skin cancer than contains melanin pigment.

Metabolism— the chemical and physical processes continuously going in the body involving the creation and breakdown of molecules.

Metastasis— the spread of a cancer from one part of the body to another. For instance lung cancer could spread to the brain or liver.

Molecule— the smallest particle of an element or compound. It is made of atoms.

Monoamine oxidase— enzymes in the brain that break down neurotransmitters, such as norepinephine, dopamine, phenylethylamine, and others. Two types are present, A and B. As we age, the activity of these enzymes increases. There is a very interesting medicine, called deprenyl or Eldepryl, that blocks the activity of MAO type B, allowing more neurotransmitters to stay and stimulate neurons.

Multiple Sclerosis— a chronic disease in which there is scattered demyelination of the central nervous system; it is characterized by speech defects, loss of muscular coordination, etc. Demyelination means loss of the protective sheath (myelin) around a nerve.

Myeloma— a malignant tumor of the bone marrow.

Natural killer cell— a type of white blood cell that can destroy viruses and cancer cells.

Neuron— a brain cell. There are over 100 billion of these cells in our brain. Neurons communicate with each other through chemicals called neurotransmitters.

Neurotransmitter— a biochemical substance, such as norepinephrine, serotonin, dopamine, phenylethylamine, acetylcholine, or endorphin, that relays messages from one neuron to another.

Optic tract (or optic nerve)— a bundle of nerves which is a continuation of the retina. It relays visual information to other parts of our brain.

Organelle— a small structure within a cell that has a specialized function. A mitochondrion is one example.

Parkinson's disease— a condition in later life involving damage to a certain part of the brain called the substantia nigra. Patients with this disease have muscular rigidity and tremor. A medicine called Eldepryl, a monoamine oxidase type B inhibitor, is helpful in treating this condition.

Pheromone— any of various chemical substances, secreted externally by certain animals, which convey information to and produce specific responses in other individuals of the same species.

Photon— the quantum energy of light, generally regarded as a discrete particle having zero mass, no electric charge, and an indefinitely long lifetime.

Pineal gland— a small gland shaped somewhat like a pine cone located in the middle of the human brain. It secretes a hormone called melatonin which influences the circadian rhythm, immune function, other hormones, and more. Light enters through our eyes and is relayed through a few bundles of nerves to the pineal gland. Light exposure stops melatonin secretion while darkness induces the pineal to make melatonin. In some lower vertebrates, the pineal is attached to a lens and retina, which shows it to be intimately associated with the evolution of eyes. The pineal detects light through the skull in some fishes, lizards, and birds. Some lizards have an opening in the skull for their pineal or "third eye." In fishes that can change color to match the background, the pineal perceives the level of light and controls the color change.

Placebo— a dummy pill that contains no active ingredient.

Prostate gland— a partly muscular gland surrounding the urethra at the base of the bladder. It secretes a lubricating fluid that is discharged with the sperm. See the diagram in chapter 10.

Receptor— a special arrangement on a cell that recognizes a molecule and interacts with it. This allows the molecule to either enter the cell or stimulate it in a specific way.

Retina— the innermost coat of cells of the back part of the eyeball. These cells are sensitive to light. They are an extension of the optic nerve which takes the image formed on the retina to the brain.

Serotonin— a brain chemical (neurotransmitter) that relays messages between brain cells (neurons). It is one of the primary mood neurotransmitters. It is derived form tryptophan, the amino acid. Serotonin can be converted to melatonin.

Serotonin reuptake inhibitor— a medicine that prevents the breakdown of serotonin, thus allowing a higher level of serotonin to be present in the brain. This often leads to an elevated mood.

Suprachiasmatic nucleus—a small section of the hypothalamus which is one of the most important regions of the brain in regulating our circadian rhythms. It has connections to the retina of the eye and the pineal gland.

Thymus— a gland located in the upper part of the chest, or the bottom part of the throat. It is involved in the development of the immune system, especially the maturation of T lymphocytes.

Triglyceride— a type of fat that circulates in the bloodstream. A glycerol molecule forms the backbone to which one, two or three fatty acids attach. High blood triglyceride levels can lead to atherosclerosis, blockage of arteries.

Tryptophan— an amino acid that needs to be ingested through foods since the body cannot manufacture it. It is converted to the neurotransmitter serotonin.

Tyrosine— an amino acid that we ingest through protein foods. It is converted to the neurotransmitters norepinephrine and dopamine.

Urethra— the canal through which urine flows out of the bladder.

References

Introduction

Maestroni G, Conti A, Pierpaoli W. *Pineal melatonin, its fundamental immunoregulatory role in aging and cancer.* Annals NY Acad Sciences 521:140-8, 1988.

Chapter One

Barchas J D, Da Costa F, Spector S. *Acute pharmacology of melatonin.* Nature 214:919-920, 1967.

Lerner A, Case J, Takahashi Y et al. *Isolation of melatonin, the pineal gland factor that lightens melanocytes.* J American Chemical Society 80:2587, 1958.

Lerner A, Nordlund J. *Melatonin: clinical pharmacology.* J Neural Trans Suppl 13:339-347, 1978. The first person given melatonin intravenously, 200 mg, for 7 days did not show evidence of delayed toxicity 18 years later.

Nickelsen T, Demisch L, Demisch K, Radermacher B, Shoffling K. *Influence of subchronic intake of melatonin at various times of the day on fatigue and hormonal levels: a placebo-controlled, double-blind trial.* J Pineal Res 6:325-34, 1989. Fifty mg of melatonin was given to 25 subjects for 1 week. Twelve pituitary and peripheral hormone levels measured did not change.

Terzolo M, Piovesan A, Puligheddu B, Torta M, Osella G, Paccotti P, Angeli A. *Effects of long-term, low-dose, time-specified melatonin administration on endocrine and cardiovascular variables in adult men.* J Pineal Res 9:113-24, 1990. Six healthy men were given 2 mg of melatonin daily at 6 pm. After 2 months, no change was found in levels or cortisol, testosterone, prolactin, and thyroid hormones.

Waldhauser F, Saletu B, Trinchard-Lugan I. *Sleep laboratory investigations on hypnotic properties of melatonin.* Psychopharmacology 100:222-6, 1990.

Voordouw B, Euser R, Verdonk R, Alberda B, de Jong F, Drogendijk A, Fauser B, Cohen M. *Melatonin and melatonin-progestin combinations alter pituitary-ovarian function in women and can inhibit ovulation.* J Clin End Metab 74:108-17, 1992.

CHAPTER TWO

Czeisler C, Dumont M, Duffy J, Steinberg J, Richardson G, Brown E, Sanchez R, Rios D, Ronda J. *Association of sleep-wake habits in older people with changes in output of circadian pacemaker.* Lancet 340:933-36, 1992.

Haimov I, Laudon M, Zisapel N, Souroujon M, Nof D, Shlitner A, Herer P, Tzischinsky O, Lavie P. *Sleep disorders and melatonin rhythms in elderly people.* British Medical Journal 309:167, 1994.

Illnerova H, Buresova M, Presl J. *Melatonin rhythm in human milk.* J Clin Endocrinol Metab 77:838-41, 1993.

Jaldo-Alba F, Munoz-Hoyos A, Molina-Carballo A, Molina-Font J, Acuna-Castroviejo D. *Light deprivation increases plasma levels of melatonin during the first 72 h of life in human infants.* Acta Endocrinologica 129:442-5, 1993.

Kloeden P, Rossler R, Rossler O. *Timekeeping in genetically programmed aging.* Experimental Gerontology 28:109-118, 1993.

Kohli et al. *Computed tomographic evaluation of pineal calcification.* Indian J Med Res 95:139-142, 1992.

Lang J, Rivest R, Schlaepfer J, Bradtke M, Aubert L, Sizonenko P. *Diurnal rhythm of melatonin action on sexual maturation of male rats.* Neuroendocrinology 38:261-268, 1984.

Nair N, Hariharasubramanian N, Pilapil C, Isaac I, Thavundayil J. *Plasma melatonin – an index of brain aging in humans?* Biol Psychiatry 21:141-150, 1986.

Prinz P, Vitiello M, Raskind M, Thorpy M. *Geriatrics: sleep disorders and aging.* N Engl J Med 323:520-6, 1990.

Reuss S, Spies C, Schroder H, Vollrath L. *The aged pineal gland: reduction in pinealocyte number and adrenergic innervation in male rats.* Exp Gerontology 25:183-188, 1990. In addition to pinealocytes becoming less efficient, there is reduced adrenergic innervation as well as falling beta adrenergic receptor density on the surface of the pinealocytes.

Rivest R, Lang U, Aubert l, Sizonenko P. *Daily administration of melatonin delays rat vaginal opening and disrupts the first estrus cycles: evidence that these effects are synchronized by the onset of light.* Endocrinology 116:779-787, 1985.

Van Coevorden A, Mockel J, Laurent E, Kerkhofs M, L'Hermite-Baleriaux M, Decoster C, Neve P, Van Cauter E. *Neuroendocrine rhythms and sleep in aging men.* Am J Physiology 260:E651-61, 1991.

Waldhauser F, Ehrhart B, Forster E. *Clinical aspects of the melatonin action: impact of development, aging, and puberty, involvement of melatonin in psychiatric disease and importance of neuroimmunoendocrine interactions.* Experientia 49:671-81, 1993.

Waldhauser F, Weiszenbacher G, Tatzer E. *Alterations in nocturnal serum melatonin levels in humans with growth and aging.*

J Clin End Metab 66:648-652, 1988.

CHAPTER THREE

Callaway, J C. *A proposed mechanism for the visions of dream sleep.* Medical Hypotheses 26:119-124, 1988.

Hardeland R, Reiter, R, Poeggeler, B, Tan, D. *The significance of the metabolism of the neurohormone melatonin: antioxidative protection and formation of bioactive substances.* Neuroscience and Biobehavioral Reviews 17:347-357, 1993.

Mirmiran M, Pevet P. *Effects of melatonin and 5-methoxy-tryptamine on sleep-wake patterns in the male rat.* J Pineal Res 3:135-41, 1986.

CHAPTER FOUR

Anisimov V, Khavinson V, Morozov V. *Twenty years of study on effects of pineal peptide preparation: Epithalamin in experimental gerontology and oncology.* Annals NY Acad Sciences 719:483-493, 1994. Chronic treatment of female C3H/Sn mice with epithalamin in a single dose, 0.5 mg, started at the age of 3.5 months, prolonged their mean life span by 40% and increased their maximum life span by 3.5 months.

Becker-Andre M, Wiesenberg I, et al. *Pineal gland hormone melatonin binds and activates an orphan of the nuclear receptor superfamily.* J Biolog Chem 269:28531-28534, 1994.

Caroleo M, Doria G, Nistico G. *Melatonin restores immunodepression in aged and cyclophosphamide-treated mice.* Annals NY Acad Sciences 719:343-352, 1994.

Hardeland R, Reiter, R, Poeggeler, B, Tan, D. *The significance of the metabolism of the neurohormone melatonin: antioxidative protection and formation of bioactive substances.* Neuroscience and Biobehavioral Reviews 17:347-357, 1993. Excellent explanation of many details of melatonin's metabolism and antioxidant effects. The 5-methoxy group, by which melatonin differs from 5-hydroxylated indoles, results in a significant increase in radical-trapping capacity.

Huether, G. *Melatonin synthesis in the gastrointestinal tract and the impact of nutritional factors on circulating melatonin.* Annals NY Acad Sciences 719:146-157, 1994. "If it is true that the anti-aging properties of melatonin are related to its ability to protect the organism against hydroxyl-radical mediated oxidative damage, food shortage and long periods of darkness would favor longevity. However, under wildlife conditions, selection pressure always favored the development of mechanisms for a maximal recruitment of food, and a life in latitudes of long darkness automatically exposes the organism to colder climates, increases energy and therefore food requirements, the rate of energy metabolism and therefore, the risk of oxidative damage. In this dilemma, evolution found a clever solution by using melatonin as a signal to inhibit reproduction. Now two different strategies could be combined: survival of the species by having a lot of offspring (due to inadequate formation of melatonin for protection of individuals under conditions of warm climates, long days and maximal food reserves) and survival of the species by extended individual lifetimes, allowing for a high degree of adaptation and transmission of learned experience from parent generations to their offspring (due to maximal production of melatonin under conditions of shorter days, colder climates and limited food reserves. Consequently, longevity could only be achieved at the expense of reproduction, and— if the scenario outlined above turns out to be true— the light- and nutrition-dependent formation of melatonin may be the secret how nature was able to achieve this goal."

Irwin M, Mascovich B, Gillin C, Willoughby R, Pike J, Smith T. *Partial sleep deprivation reduces natural killer cell activity in humans.* Psychosom Med 56:493-8, 1994.

Kloeden P, Rossler R, Rossler O. *Timekeeping in genetically programmed aging.* Experimental Gerontology 28:109-118, 1993. The nightly melatonin peak changes with age, thus providing a potential signal to inform all of the cells of an organism of its age. This article proposes that the decoding of this 'durational signal' at the cellular level is carried out with the aid of the sleep induced pCO2 changes in the blood.

Kloeden P. *Does a centralized clock for aging exist?* Gerontology 36:314-322, 1990.

Lesnikov V, Pierpaoli W. *Pineal cross-transplantation (old-to-young and vice versa) as evidence for an endogenous "aging clock."* Annals NY Acad Sciences 719:456- 460, 1994.

Lopez-Gongalez M, Calvo J, Segura J, Guerrero J. *Characterization of melatonin binding sites in human peripheral blood neutrophils.* Biotech Therap 4:253-62, 1993.

Maestroni G, Conti A, Pierpaoli W. *Pineal melatonin, its fundamental immunoregulatory role in aging and cancer.* Annals NY Acad Sciences 521:140-8, 1988.

Maestroni G, Conti A, Pierpaoli W. *Role of the pineal gland in immunity. Circadian synthesis and release of melatonin modulates the antibody response and antagonizes the immunosuppressive effect of corticosterone.* J Neuroimmun 3:19-30, 1986.

Maestroni G. *The immunoendocrine role of melatonin.* J Pineal Res 14:1-10, 1993. The immunoenhancing action of melatonin seems to be mediated by T-helper cell-derived opioid peptides as well as by lymphokines and perhaps, by pituitary hormones. Melatonin-induced-immuno-opioids and lymphokines imply the presence of specific binding sites of melatonin receptors on cells of the immune system. On the other hand, lymphokines such as gamma-interferon and interleukin-2 as well as thymic hormones can modulate the synthesis of melatonin in the pineal gland. The pineal gland night thus be viewed as the crux of a sophisticated immunoneuroendocrine network which functions as an unconscious, diffuse sensory organ.

Malm O, Skaug O, Lingjaerde P. *The effect of pinealectomy on bodily growth, survival rate and P32 uptake in the rat.* Acta Endocrinol 30:22-28, 1959.

Mocchegiani E, Bulian D, Santarelli L, Tibaldi A, Pierpaoli W, Fabris N. *The zinc-melatonin interrelationship, a working hypothesis.* Annals NY Acad Sciences 719:298-307, 1994.

Morrey K, McLachlan J, Serkin C, Bakouche O. *Activation of human monocytes by the pineal hormone melatonin.* J Immunology 153:2671-80, 1994. Melatonin activates monocytes and induces their cytotoxic properties, along with IL-1 secretion.

Pierpaoli W, Dall'ara A, Pedrinis E, Regelson W. *The pineal control of aging: the effects of melatonin and pineal grafting on the survival of older mice.* Annals NY Acad Sciences 621:291-313, 1991.

Pierpaoli W, Regelson W. *Pineal control of aging: effect of melatonin and pineal grafting on aging mice.* Proc Nat Acad Sci 91:787-91, 1994. Fifteen month old BALB/c strain female mice given melatonin lived up to 28 months compared to 24 for controls.

Pierrefiche G, Topall G, Courboin G, Henriet I, Laborit H. *Antioxidant activity of melatonin in mice.* Res Commun Chem Pathol Pharmacol 80:211-23, 1993.

Poon A, Liu Z, Pang C, Brown G, Pang S. *Evidence for a direct action of melatonin on the immune system.* Biolog Signals 3:107-17, 1994. Melatonin receptors were found on lymphoid tissues.

Puigdevall V, Laudo C, Elosegui L, Del Rio M, San Martin L, Escanero J. *Hypothalamic and pineal concentrations of magnesium and calcium after a sustained administration of melatonin.*

J Endocrinol Invest 16 (Suppl 1 to no. 8):253, 1993. Rats injected with melatonin every day showed reduction in pineal calcium concentrations. Could melatonin supplementation result in less pineal calcium deposition?

Reiter R, Tan D, Poeggeler B, Menendez-Pelaez A, Chen L, Saarela S. *Melatonin as a free radical scavenger: Implications for aging and age-related diseases.* Annals NY Acad Sciences 721:1-12, 1994. "Melatonin is wide spread in the animal kingdom. Indeed, it may be produced in all aerobic organisms. For example, a circadian rhythm of melatonin has been found in a dinoflagellate, Gonyaulax polyedra, which closely resembles the melatonin cycle in the blood of humans. It also seems likely that most, if to all, species between algae and humans produce melatonin for antioxidant protection. Indeed, we are currently working under the assumption that melatonin evolved coincident with aerobic metabolism to specifically protect cells and organs from the resulting oxidative attack by oxygen centered radicals. It is also our opinion that the other function so melatonin (e.g. regulation of season reproduction and circadian rhythmicity), which seemingly rely on membrane-bound receptors, evolved at a much later date. This speculation is supported by the physicochemical properties of melatonin."

Reiter R. *Interactions of the pineal hormone melatonin with oxygen-centered free radicals: a brief review.* Brazilian J Med Biological Res 26:1141-55, 1993.

Reiter R. *Pineal function during aging: attenuation of the melatonin rhythm and its neurobiological consequences.* Acto Neuro Experimentalis 54(Suppl.):31-39, 1994. Excellent article, easy read.

Reppert S, Weaver D, Ebisawa T. *Cloning and characterization of a mammalian melatonin receptor that mediates reproductive and circadian responses.* Neuron 13:1177-1185, 1994.

Stankov B, Gervasoni M, Scaglione F, Perego R, Cova D, Mara-bini L, Fraschini F. *Primary pharmaco-toxicological evaluation of 2-iodomelatonin, a potent melatonin agonist.* Life Sciences 53:1357-1365, 1993.

Stokkan K, Reiter R, Nonaka K. *Food restriction retards aging of the pineal gland.* Brain Research 545:66-72, 1991.

Sze S, Liu W, Ng T. *Stimulation of murine splenocytes by mela-tonin and methoxytryptamine.* J Neural Transmission Gen Sect 94:115-26, 1993. Male mice received melatonin and methoxytrypt-amine in the drinking water for 2 weeks. Splenocytes from mela-tonin treated mice showed an augmented mitogenic response to concanavalin A and lipopolysaccharide while splenocytes from methoxytryptamine-treated mice demonstrated an enhance mito-genic response to lipopolysaccharide.

Tan D, Reiter R, Chen L, Poeggeler B. Manchester L, Barlow-Walden L. *Both physiological and pharmacological levels of mela-tonin reduce DNA adduct formation induced by the carcinogen safrole.* Carcinogenesis 15:215-218, 1994.

CHAPTER FIVE

MacFarlane J, Cleghorn J, Brown G, Streiner D. *The effects of exogenous melatonin on the total sleep time and daytime alertness of chronic insomniacs: a preliminary study.* Biological Psychiatry 30:371-376, 1991.

Biochemicals— Organic Compounds for Research and Diag-nostic Reagents, Sigma Chemical Co., St. Louis, MO, p635, 1993. This reference recommends storage of melatonin in the refrigera-tor, and was provided by Vitamin Research Products, Carson City, Nevada.

CHAPTER SIX

Insomnia

Arendt J, Bojkowski C, Franey C, Wright J, Marks V. *Immunoassay of 6-hydroxymelatonin sulfate in human plasma and urine: Abolition of the 24-hour rhythm with atenolol.* J Clin Endocrinology Metab 60:1166-1173, 1985. Pineal cells (pinealocytes) have beta receptors on their membranes. Stimulation of these beta receptors by norepinephrine induces melatonin release. When these beta receptors are blocked by medicines such as propranolol or atenolol, melatonin production decreases or stops.

Dahlitz M, Alvarez B, Vignau J, English J, Arendt J, Parkes J. *Delayed sleep phase syndrome response to melatonin.* Lancet 337: 1121-24, 1991.

Ekman A, Leppaluoto J, Huttunen P, Aranko K, Vakkuri O. *Ethanol inhibits melatonin secretion in healthy volunteers in a dose-dependent randomized double blind cross-over study.* J Clin Endocrin and Metab 77:780-3, 1993.

Ferrini-Strambi L, Zucconi M, Biella G, Stankov B, Fraschini F, Oldani A, Smirne S. *Effect of melatonin on sleep microstructure: preliminary results in healthy subjects.* Sleep 16:744-7, 1993.

Jan J, Espezel H. *Melatonin treatment of chronic sleep disorders.* Developmental Medicine and Child Neurology 37:279-280, 1995.

Laakso M, Hatonen T, Stenberg D, Alila A, Smith S. *One-hour exposure to moderate illuminance (500 lux) shifts the human melatonin rhythm.* J Pineal Res 15:21-6, 1993.

MacFarlane J, Cleghorn J, Brown G, Streiner D. *The effects of exogenous melatonin on the total sleep time and daytime alertness of chronic insomniacs: a preliminary study.* Biological Psychiatry 30:371-376, 1991.

Monteleone P, D'Istria M, De Luca B, Serino I, Maj M, Kemali

D. *Pineal response to isoproterenol in rats chronically treated with electroconvulsive shock*. Brain Research Bulletin 32:237-9, 1993. Chronic stress through electroconvulsive shock (ECS) treatment affects beta 1 receptor-mediated melatonin production in the pineal gland. Further studies need to elucidate whether the blunted melatonin response to isoproterenol in these ECS-treated rats is due to a downregulation of pinealocyte beta-adrenergic receptors.

Murphy P, Badia P, Myers B, Boecker M, Wright K. *Nonsteroidal anti-inflammatory drugs affect normal sleep patterns in humans*. Physiology and Behavior, 55:1063-6, 1994.

Zhao Z, Touitou Y. *Kinetic changes of melatonin release in rat pineal perfusions at different circadian stages. Effects of corticosteroids*. Acta Endocrinol (Copenhagen) 129:81-8, 1993.

Jet Lag

Claustrat B, Brun J, David M, Sassolas G, Chazot G. *Melatonin and jet lag: confirmatory result using a simplified protocol*. Biological Psychiatry 32:705-11, 1992. Melatonin supplements taken the evening of sleep in the new time zone significantly helped adjustment to sleep.

Harma M, Laitinen J, Partinen M, Suvanto S. *The effect of four-day round trip flights over 10 time zones on the circadian variation of salivary melatonin and cortisol in airline flight attendants*. Ergonomics 37:1479-1489, 1993.

Petrie K, Dawson A, Thompson L, Brook R. *A double-blind trial of melatonin as a treatment for jet lag in international cabin crew*. Biological Psychiatry 33:526-30, 1993.

Shift Work

Eastman C, Stewart K, Mahoney M, Liu L, Fogg L. *Dark goggles and bright light improve circadian rhythm adaptation to nightshift work*. Sleep 17:535-543, 1994.

Folkard S, Arendt J, Clark M. *Can melatonin improve shift workers' tolerance of the night shift? Some preliminary findings.* Chronobiology International 10:315-20, 1993.

Mood

Carmen J, Post R, Buswell R, et al. *Negative effects of melatonin on depression.* Am J Psychiatry 140:292-304, 1982.

Neville K, McNaughton N. *Anxiolytic-like action of melatonin on acquisition but not performance of DRL.* Pharm Biochem Beh 24:1497-1502, 1986. Melatonin shares some anxiolytic properties of chlodiazepoxide (Librium). Melatonin inhibits diazepam binding, suggesting that it interacts directly or indirectly, with the benzodiazepine receptor. Melatonin increases GABA levels, so do anxiolytic drugs. It can potentiate barbiturate-induced sleep time. It can also act as an anticonvulsant.

Petterborg L, Thalen B, Kjellman B, Wetterberg L. *Effect of melatonin replacement on serum hormone rhythms in a patient lacking endogenous melatonin.* Brain Research Bulletin 27:181-5, 1991. The authors also found melatonin administration produced robust nocturnal peaks in serum growth hormone and prolactin levels.

Pierrefiche G, Zerbib R, Laborit H. *Anxiolytic activity of melatonin in mice: involvement of benzodiazepine receptors.* Res Commun Chem Pathol Pharmacol 82:131-42, 1993.

Totterdell P, Reynolds S, Parkinson B, Briner R. *Associations of sleep with everyday mood, minor symptoms and social interaction experience.* Sleep 17:466-475, 1994.

CHAPTER SEVEN

Arendt J, Bhanji S, Franey C, Mattingly D. *Plasma melatonin levels in anorexia nervosa.* British J Psychiatry 161:361-4, 1992.

Aronson B, Bell-Pedersen D, Block G, Bos N, et al. *Circadian Rhythms*. Brain Research Reviews, 18:315-333, 1993. A thorough and detailed review of the role of the suprachiasmatic nucleus. The SCN receives visual signals from eyes directly via the reticulohypothalamic tract and indirectly via the geniculohypothalamic tract; they then transmit the integrated signal to the pineal gland via the upper thoracic cord and superior cervical ganglia of the peripheral sympathetic nervous system.

Cagnacci A, Soldani R, Yen S. *The effect of light on core body temperature is mediated by melatonin in women.* J Clin Endo Met 76:1036-8, 1993.

Huether G, Poeggeler B, Reimer A, George A. *Effect of tryptophan administration on circulating melatonin levels in chicks and rats: Evidence for stimulation of melatonin synthesis and release in the gastrointestinal tract.* Life Sciences 51:945-953, 1992. Administration of L-tryptophan to rats and chicks causes a rapid and dose-dependent elevation of melatonin. Partial ligature of the portal vein almost abolished circulating melatonin. The tryptophan-induced increase of melatonin in the portal blood preceded the increase in the systemic circulation. The enterochromaffin cells of the gastrointestinal tract appear to be the major source of the tryptophan-inducing rise of circulating melatonin.

Laakso M, Hatonen T, Stenberg D, Alila A, Smith S. *One-hour exposure to moderate illuminance (500 lux) shifts the human melatonin rhythm.* J Pineal Res 15:21-6, 1993.

Lee P, Pang S. *Melatonin and its receptors in the gastrointestinal tract.* Biological Signals 2:181-93, 1993.

Levine M, Milliron A, Duffy L. *Diurnal and seasonal rhythms of melatonin, cortisol and testosterone in interior Alaska.* Arctic Medical Research 53:25-34, 1994.

Nowak J, Zurawska E, Zawilska J. *Melatonin and its generat-*

ing system in vertebrate retina: circadian rhythm, effect of environmental lighting and interaction with dopamine. Neurochem Int 14:397-406, 1989.

Pang C, Brown G, Tang P, Cheng K, Pang S. *2-[125 I] iodomelatonin binding sites in the lung and heart: a link between the photoperiodic signal, melatonin, and the cardiopulmonary system.* Biological Signals 2:228-36, 1993.

Panza J, Epstein S, Quyyumi A. *Circadian variation in vascular tone and its relation to alpha-sympathetic vasoconstrictor activity.* N England J Med 325:986-90, 1991.

Reiter R, Tan D, Poeggeler B, Menendez-Pelaez A, Chen L, Saarela S. *Melatonin as a free radical scavenger: Implications for aging and age-related diseases.* Annals NY Acad Sciences 721:1-12, 1994.

Reiter R. *Electromagnetic fields and melatonin production.* Biomedicine and Pharmacotherapy 47:439-44, 1993. Exposure of non-human mammals to sinusoidal electric and/or magnetic fields often reduces pineal melatonin production.

Reiter, R. News Physiol Sci 6:223-227, 1991. The nightly formation of melatonin is primarily a result of the release of norepinephrine (NE) from postganglionic sympathetic neurons ending in the pineal gland. Once released, NE interacts with beta-adrenergic receptors linked via a G-stimulatory protein to adenylate cyclase in the membrane of the pinealocytes. Activation of adenylate cyclase increases intracellular cAMP production, which leads to the induction of N-acetyltransferase (NAT), the rate limiting enzyme in melatonin synthesis. About 85% of the melatonin formed in the pineal gland seems to be a result of NE interaction with beta-receptors. About 15% of the melatonin produced seems to result from the adrenergic stimulation of alpha-adrenergic receptors. The melatonin rhythm is progressively attenuated during aging, presumably due to a reduction in the number of beta-adrenergic receptors in the pinealocyte membranes.

Saarela S, Reiter R: *Functions of melatonin in thermoregulatory processes.* Life Sciences 54:295-311, 1993. Excellent review. Light stops the secretion of a brain chemical called norepinephrine into the pineal gland. When there is no light, norepinephrine is released and this stimulates the pineal cells to produce melatonin. Melatonin is involved in circadian body temperature adjustments.

Stokkan D, Reiter R. *Melatonin rhythms in Arctic urban residents.* J Pineal Res 16:33-6, 1994.

Strassman R, Qualls C, Lisansky J, Peake G. *Elevated rectal temperature produced by all-night bright light is reversed by melatonin infusion in men.* J Applied Physiology 71:2178-2182, 1991.

Tamarkin, Baird B, Ammelda O. *Melatonin: a coordinating signal for mammalian reproduction?* Science 227:714-20, 1985.

CHAPTER EIGHT

Aschoff J. *The timing of defecation within the sleep-wake cycle of humans during temporal isolation.* J Biological Rhythms 9:43-50, 1994.

Czeisler C, Shanahan R, Klerman E, Martens J, Brotman A, Emens J, Klein T, Rizzo J. *Suppression of melatonin secretion in some blind patients by exposure to bright light.* N England J Med 332:6-11, 1995.

Sack R, et al: *Circadian rhythm abnormalities in totally blind people; incidence and clinical significance.* J Clin Endocrinol Metab 75:127-34, 1992.

Sack R, Lewy, A. *Human circadian rhythms: lessons from the blind.* Ann Med 25:303-5, 1993.

Sandyk R. *Melatonin and maturation of REM sleep.* Int J Neuroscience 63:105-14, 1992.

Waldhauser F, Saletu B, Trinchard-Lugan I. *Sleep laboratory investigations on hypnotic properties of melatonin.* Psychopharmacology 100:222-6, 1990.

CHAPTER NINE

Bootzin R, Perlis M. *Nonpharmacological treatments of insomnia.* J Clin Psychiatry 53(6, suppl):37-41, 1992.

Deacon S, Arendt J. *Phase-shifts in melatonin, 6-sulphatoxymelatonin and alertness rhythms after treatment with moderately bright light at night.* Clinical Endocrinology 40:413-20, 1994.

Doghramji K. *Causes, pathogenesis, and management of sleep disorders.* Compr Ther 16:49-59, 1990.

Ekman A, Leppaluoto J, Huttunen P, Aranko K, Vakkuri O. *Ethanol inhibits melatonin secretion in healthy volunteers in a dose-dependent randomized double blind cross-over study.* J Clinical Endocrinology and Metabolism 77:780-3, 1993.

Lemmer B, Bruhl T, Witte K, Pflug B, Kohler W, Touitou Y. *Effects of bright light on circadian patterns of cyclic adenosine monophosphate, melatonin and cortisol in healthy subjects.* European J Endocrinology 130:472-7, 1994.

Monteleone P, Maj M, Fusco M, Orazzo C, Kemali D. *Physical exercise at night blunts the nocturnal increase of plasma melatonin levels in healthy humans.* Life Sciences 47:1989-95, 1990.

Myers B, Badia P. *Immediate effects of different light intensities on body temperature and alertness.* Physiology and Behavior 54:199-202, 1993.

Van Reeth O, Sturis J, et al. *Nocturnal exercise phase delays circadian rhythms of melatonin and thyrotropin secretion in normal men.* Am J Physiology 266:E964-974, 1994.

CHAPTER TEN

Pozo D, Reiter R, Calvo J, Guerrero J. *Physiological concentrations of melatonin inhibit nitric oxide synthase in rat cerebellum.* Life Sciences 55:455-460, 1994.

Cholesterol

Aoyama H, Mori N, Mori W. Atherosclerosis 69:269-272, 1988.

Muller-Wieland D, Behnke B, Koopman, D, Krone, W. *Melatonin inhibits LDL receptor activity and cholesterol synthesis in freshly isolated human mononuclear leukocytes.* Biochemical and Biophysical Research Communications, 203:416-21, 1994.

Prostate

Horst H, Buck A, Adam K. *Orally administered melatonin stimulates the 3 alpha/beta hydroxy steroid oxidoreductase but not the 5 alpha reductase in the ventral prostate and seminal vesicles of pinealectomized rats.* Experientia 38:968-970, 1982.

Shirima K, Furuya T, Takeo Y, Shimizu K, Maekawa K. *Direct effect of melatonin on the accesory sexual organs in pinealectomized male rats kept in constant darkness.* J Endocrinol 95:87-94, 1982.

Sriuilai W, Withyacitumroarnku B. *Stereological changes in rat ventral prostate induced by melatonin.* J Pineal Res 6:111-119, 1989.

Osteoporosis

Machida M, Dubousset J, Imamura Y, Iwaya T, Yamada T, Kimura J. *Role of melatonin deficiency in the development of scoliosis in pinealectomized chickens.* J Bone Joint Surg (Br) 77-B:134-8, 1995.

Sandyk R, Anastasiadis P, Anninos P, Tsagas N. *Is postmenopausal osteoporosis related to pineal gland functions?* Internat J Neurosci 62:215-25, 1992.

Immunity

Caroleo M, Frasca D, Nistico G, Doria G. *Melatonin as immunomodulator in immunodeficient mice.* Immunopharmac 23:81-9, 1992.

Cancer

Aldeghi R, Lissoni P, Barni S, Ardizzolia A, Tancini G, Piperno A, Pozzi M, Ricci G, Conti A, Maestroni G. *Low-dose interleukin-2 subcutaneous immunotherapy in association with the pineal hormone melatonin as a first-line therapy in locally advanced or metastatic hepatocellular carcinoma.* European J Cancer 30A:167-170, 1994. Good results with melatonin and IL-2 therapy.

Bartsch C, Bartsch H, Fluchter S, Mecke D, Lippert T. *Diminished pineal function coincides with disturbed circadian endocrine rhythmicity in untreated primary cancer patients. Consequence of premature aging or of tumor growth.* Annals NY Acad Sciences 719:502-525, 1994.

Bartsch H, Bartsch C, Simon W, Flehmig B, Ebels I, Lippert T. *Antitumor activity of the pineal gland: effect of unidentified substances versus the effect of melatonin.* Oncology 49:27-30, 1992.

Coleman N, Reiter R. *Breast cancer, blindness, and melatonin.* Eur J Cancer 28:501-3, 1992.

Crespo D, Fernandez-Viadero C, Verduga R, Ovejero V, Cos S. *Interaction between melatonin and estradiol on morphological and morphometric features of MCF-7 human breast cancer cells.* J Pineal Res 16:215-22, 1994

Gonzalez R, Sanchez A, Ferguson J, Balmer C, Daniel C, Cohn A, Robinson W. *Melatonin therapy of advanced human malignant melanoma.* Melanoma Res 1:237-43, 1991.

Hill S, Blask D. *Effect of the pineal hormone melatonin on the proliferation and morphological characteristics of human breast cancer cells (MCF7) in culture.* Cancer Research 48:6121-6126,

1988.

Lissoni P, Barni S, Ardizzoia A, Tancini G, Conti A, Maestroni G. *A randomized study with the pineal hormone melatonin versus supportive care alone in patients with brain metastases due to solid neoplasms.* Cancer 73:699-701, 1994.

Lissoni P, Barni S, Cattaneo G, Tancini G, Esposti G, Esposti D. *Clinical results with the pineal hormone melatonin in advanced cancer resistant to standard antitumor therapies.* 48:448-450, 1991.

Lissoni P, Barni S, Tancini G, Ardizzoia A, Ricci G, Aldeghi R, et al. *A randomized study with subcutaneous low-dose interleukin 2 alone vs. interleukin 2 plus the pineal neurohormone melatonin in advanced solid neoplams other than renal cancer and melanoma.* British J Cancer 69:196-199, 1994. Eighty patients with locally advanced or metastatic solid tumors were divided into two groups. One group received interleukin 2 (IL-2), and the other group received IL-2 with the addition of melatonin 40 mg each night at 8 pm. Those receiving melatonin had a significantly better response.

Lissoni P, Ardizzoia A, et al. *Amplification of eosinophilia by melatonin during the immunotherapy of cancer with interleukin-2.* J Bio Regulators and Homeostatic Agents 7:34-36, 1993. The immune system uses many different mechanisms to prevent the development of tumors and to limit their growth. The varied types of immune cells involved in this process include *lymphocytes, natural killer cells, macrophages, eosinophils,* and more. Eosinophils have recently been found to help fight cancer cells. Higher levels of eosinophils have been found in those whose cancer is going into regression. In this study 30 patients with advanced forms of cancer received interleukin-2, a natural chemical which fights cancer cells. Sixteen of these patients received IL-2 alone while the other 14 received IL-2 in addition to 10 mg of melatonin orally at night. Patients who received melatonin had significantly more eosinophils in their bloodstream. The researchers believe that this may result in improving the ability of the body to fight off the cancer.

Lissoni, P, Barni S, Tancini G, Ardizzoia A, Brivio F, et al. *Therapeutic use of the pineal hormone melatonin in human neoplasms: update results.* Acta Neurobiologiae Experimentalis. 54 (Suppl.):127-8, 1994.

Neri B, Fiorelli C, Moroni F, Nicita G, Paoletti M, Ponchietti R, Raugei A, Santoni G, Trippitelli A, Grechi G. *Modulation of human lymphoblastoid interferon activity by melatonin in metastatic renal cell carcinoma. A phase II study.* Cancer 73:3015-9, 1994. Twenty-two patients with documented progression of renal cell carcinoma entered a trial in which the authors studied the effect of a long-term regimen (12 months) with human lymphoblastoid interferon (IFN), 3 mega units (MU) intramuscularly 3 times per week, and melatonin, 10 mg orally every day. There were seven remissions (33%), three complete, involving lung and soft tissue and four partial, with a median duration at the time of the writing of 16 months. Nine patients achieved stable disease, and five progressed. General toxicity was mild.

Philo R, Berkowitz, A. *Inhibition of dunning tumor growth by melatonin.* J Urology 139:1099-1102, 1988.

Subramanian A, Kothari L. *Melatonin, a suppresser of spontaneous murine mammary tumors.* J Pineal Res 10:136-40, 1991.

Sze S, Ng T, Liu W. *Antiproliferative effect of pineal indoles on cultured tumor cell lines.* J Pineal Res 14:27-33, 1993. Methoxytryptamine and melatonin were effective in inhibiting the proliferation of several cell lines including melanoma, sarcoma, macrophage-like cell line, fibroblasts and choriocarcinoma.

Wilson S, Blask D, Lemus-Wilson, A. *Melatonin augments the sensitivity of MCF-7 human breast cancer cells to tamoxifen in vitro.* J Clin Endo Met 75:669-70, 1992.

Epilepsy

Anton-Tay F. *Melatonin: effects on brain function.* Adv Biochem Psychopharmacol 11:315-24, 1974.

Golombek D et al. *Time-dependent anticonvulsant activity of melatonin in hamsters.* Eur J Pharmacol 210:253-8, 1992.

Schapel G, Beran R, Kennaway D, McLoughney J, Matthews C. *Melatonin response in active epilepsy.* Epilepsia 36(1):75-78, 1995.

CAUTION

Diaz Lopez B, Marin Fernandez M. *Effects of melatonin administration to rats upon different parameters of the offspring.* Reproduction 7:1:7, 1983. Dosage used was 250 mcg/ml by intraperitoneal injection. The testes weight of the sons was not affected.

Hansson I, Holmdahl R, Mattsson R. *The pineal hormone melatonin exaggerates development of collagen-induced arthritis in mice.* J Neuroimmunol 39:23-30, 1992.

Kauppila et al. *Inverse seasonal relationship between melatonin and ovarian activity in humans in a region with a strong seasonal contrast in luminosity.* J Clin Endocrin Metab, 1987; 65:823-828. In humans, melatonin is believed to inhibit the release of hormones that influence the ovaries. During periods of high melatonin secretion, such as during the long, dark Arctic winter, a lower incidence of ovulatory cycles and twin pregnancies occurs.

Ooi V, Ng T. *Histological studies on the effects of pineal 5-methoxyindoles on the reproductive organs of the male golden hamster.* J Pineal Res 7(4):315-24, 1989. Melatonin injections caused a reduction in the diameters of seminiferous tubules and an inhibition of spermatogenesis. Testicular regression ranged from a decrease in the abundance of late spermatids and mature spermatozoa in some animals to an almost complete loss of spermatogenesis in others. Sertoli cells were more resistant to the treatment than other cellular components of the seminiferous tubules.

Leydig cells were reduced in size, showed a great reduction in cytoplasm, and possessed shrunken and angular nuclei.

Oxenkrug G, McIntyre I, McCauley R, Yuwiler A. *Effect of selective monoamine oxidase inhibitors on rat pineal melatonin synthesis in vitro.* J Pineal Res 5:99-109, 1988. High amounts of MAO-B inhibitors, such as deprenyl, also increase melatonin levels.

Persengiev S, Kyurkchiev S. *Selective effect of melatonin on the proliferation of lymphoid cells.* Int J Biochemistry 25:441-444, 1993. Administration of 200 microM melatonin in vitro inhibited significantly the incorporation of (3H) thymidine into both normal mouse and human lymphocytes and T-lymphoblastoid cell lines. On the contrary, melatonin provoked an increase of myeloma cell proliferation. The influence of melatonin on hybridoma cell lines was negligible. Collectively, these data demonstrated that the chief pineal indole affected selectively the processes of lymphoblastoid cell growth.

Persengiev S, Kehajova J. *Inhibitory action of melatonin and structurally related compounds on testosterone production by mouse Leydig cells in vitro.* Cell Biochem Funct 9(4):281-6, 1991. Natural indoles that are synthesized in the pineal gland and their halogenized derivatives are capable of influencing directly testosterone production by Leydig cells. Also, these results demonstrated that melatonin exerts its remarkable antigonadotrphic effects, at least in part, through the direct decrease of testosterone production.

Raynaud F, Miguel J, Vivien-Roels B, Masson-Pevet M, Pevet P. *The effect of 5-methoxytryptamine on golden hamster gonads is not a consequence of its acetylation into melatonin.* J Endocrinology 121(3):507-12, 1989. After 8 weeks of injections, 5-methoxytryptamine induced total testicular regression, while melatonin induced partial atrophy.

Silman R. *Melatonin: a contraceptive for the nineties.* European J Obstetrics, Gynecology, Reproductive Bio 49:3-9, 1993. "The hypothalamic GnRH pulse generator activates the pituitary-gonadal reproductive axis, and contraceptive techniques have advanced to the point where GnRH analogues can block this effect. However, nature has an even finer form of contraception, whereby the GnRH pulse generator is activated or inactivated at different seasons of the year through the longer duration of melatonin released in winter. A melatonin based contraceptive is undergoing phase III clinical trials."

Skene D, Bojkowski C, Arendt J. *Comparison of the effects of acute fluvoxamine (Luvox) and desipramine administration on melatonin and cortisol production in humans.* British J Clin Pharm 37:181-6, 1994. Both fluvoxamine and desipramine (Norpramin) increased nocturnal plasma melatonin concentrations. Desipramine is known to increase noradrenaline availability which induces melatonin production. Fluvoxamine inhibited the metabolism of melatonin. Fluvoxamine significantly delayed the offset time and desipramine significantly advanced the onset time of melatonin release. That the drug treatments significantly affected different aspects of the nocturnal plasma melatonin profile suggests that the amplitude of the melatonin rhythm may depend upon serotonin availability and/or melatonin metabolism whilst the onset of melatonin production depends upon noradrenaline availability.

APPENDIX

Booker, J, Hellekson, C. *Prevalence of seasonal affective disorder in Alaska.* Am J Psychiatry 149:1176-1182, 1992.

Danilenko K, Putilov A, Russkikh G, Duffy L, Ebbesson S. *Diurnal and seasonal variations of melatonin and serotonin in women with seasonal affective disorder.* Arctic Medical Research, 53:137-45, 1994.

Gazzah N, Gharib A, Delton I, Moliere P, Durand G, Christon R, Lagarde M, Sarda N. *Effect of an n-3 fatty acid-deficient diet on the adenosine-dependent melatonin release in cultured rat pineal.* J Neurochem 61:1057-63, 1993.

Harris, S, Dawson-Hughes, B. *Seasonal mood changes in 250 normal women.* Psychiatry Research, 1993; 49:77-87

Levine M, Milliron A, Duffy L. *Diurnal and seasonal rhythms of melatonin, cortisol and testosterone in interior Alaska.* Arctic Medical Research 53:25-34, 1994.

McElhinney D, Hoffman S, Robinson W, Ferguson J. *Effect of melatonin on human skin color.* J Invest Dermatol 102:258-9, 1994.

Nordlund J, Lerner A. *The effects of oral melatonin on skin color and on the release of pituitary hormones.* J Clin End Metab 45:768, 1977.

Rosenthal N. Sack D, Jacobsen F, James S, Parry B, Arendt J, Tamarkin L, Wehr T. *Melatonin in seasonal affective disorder and phototherapy.* J Neural Transm Suppl 21:257-267, 1986.

Schlager D. *Early-morning administration of short-acting beta blockers for treatment of winter depression.* Am J Psychiatry 151:1383-1385, 1994.

Wirz-Justice A, Graw P, Krauchi K, Gisin B, Arendt J, Aldhous M, Poldinger W. *Morning or night-time melatonin is ineffective in seasonal affective disorder.* J Psychiatric Research 24:129-137, 1990. Five mg of melatonin whether given at 7 am or 11 pm for a week did not improve symptoms. Light remains the therapy of choice.

INDEX

BE HAPPIER STARTING NOW

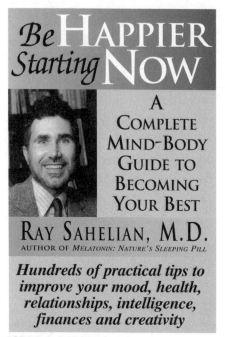

Be **HAPPIER** *Starting* **NOW**

A
COMPLETE
MIND-BODY
GUIDE TO
BECOMING
YOUR BEST

RAY SAHELIAN, M.D.

AUTHOR OF *MELATONIN: NATURE'S SLEEPING PILL*

Hundreds of practical tips to improve your mood, health, relationships, intelligence, finances and creativity

- Proven ways to start feeling better immediately
- A complete approach to living longer
- Setting and achieving goals
- Secrets of pleasure fulfillment
- The ideal diet for hapiness
- How to forgive yourself...and everyone else
- How to find meaning in life
- How to cultivate a sense of connection with yourself, others, nature, and more
- Six supplements that improve mood

ISBN 0-9639755-6-0
200 pages, 6"×9", softcover
Third printing July, 1995, new cover

"*Be Happier* will rest on your nightstand for ages. You will read it again and again, each time discovering more depth and wisdom. Dr. Ray Sahelian has delicately interlaced the poetry, spirit, and science of happiness. Open the beautiful cover and explore a land where you, everyone, mind, mood, and heart are one."
– *Arnold Fox, M.D., best-selling author of* The Beverly Hills Medical Diet *and* Immune for Life

"With a smile and an open heart, the riches in your life will increase. If a book can make you happier, when does the reading begin?"
– *Arlene Schindler,* Whole Life Times

Do you know how happy you are? Take Dr. Ray Sahelian's happiness quiz and find out. You will be certain to get new insights about yourself.

For your autographed copy of *Be Happier*, send a $15.00 check or money order (includes shipping; California residents add 99¢ tax for a total of $15.99) to:

Be Happier Press
P.O. Box 12619
Marina Del Rey, CA 90295.

To order your autographed copy of *Melatonin: Nature's Sleeping Pill*, send a $16.95 check or money order (includes shipping; California residents add $1.15 tax, for a total of $18.10) to the above address.

To order both *Melatonin: Nature's Sleeping Pill* and *Be Happier Starting Now*, send a $31.95 check or money order (includes shipping; California residents add $2.47 tax, for a total of $34.42). **Be sure to include your name and mailing address.** Orders are shipped promptly.

For a non-autographed copy, have your credit card ready and call **1-800-507-2665** to order either or both books now. Orders are shipped the same day.

You may also find both books in any bookstore. If not available, have them order through PDS (Publisher's Distribution Service) at **1-800-345-0096** or any wholesaler.

Dr. Sahelian is very much interested in your personal experience with melatonin. Please write to him at the above address or, via email, at dr.ray@ix.netcom.com. If possible include your name, age, occupation, approximately how many doses you've taken, how often you use melatonin, how long you've used it, and whether you've had any positive or negative effects. All letters will be answered if SASE is included. All email will be acknowledged.

NOTES